Free to Eat

A practical guide to reducing the symptoms
of histamine, sulphur, glutamate
and salicylate sensitivity

By Janine Lattimore
Copyright 2015 Janine Lattimore
Distributed by Amazon.com
Fifth Edition
(Re-edited and amended 2021)

Published by
Janine Lattimore
Christchurch, New Zealand
Email: info@janinelattimore.com
Web: janinelattimore.com

Copyright © 2015 Janine Kaye Lattimore

All rights reserved. No part of this publication may be reproduced or distributed in any form or by any means without written permission of the publisher, except in the case of a brief quotation embodied in critical articles and reviews.

The content of this book reflects the work and thought of the author. Every effort has been made to publish reliable and accurate information herein, but the publisher is not responsible for the validity of the information or for any outcomes resulting from the reliance thereon.

ISBN-13: 978-1521400777

Dedication

This book is dedicated to the many wonderful fellow chemical sensitivity sufferers who have researched, trialled, debated, shared and supported via numerous online forums, Facebook pages and personal blogs. The information you provided was often so helpful and even just knowing that I was not alone with my seemingly crazy reactions helped to make things tolerable when I began to despair. I deeply appreciate the hope and knowledge you have freely given. I also want to give special thanks to:

- The Food Intolerance Network Canterbury especially its wonderful coordinator Robin Fisher and members Jewel and Catherine who helped me to edit this book

- My dietitian Clarice Hebblethwaite for her advice and support

- Sue Dengate and her husband for their book Fed Up. This was the first book on salicylate intolerance I read after I learned that I suffered from it and I literally cried as I read some of the stories in the book. I am profoundly grateful to Sue and her husband for their research, lobbying and provision of information regarding chemicals in food and their effect on our mental and physical health.

- Yasmina Ykelenstam and her very informative blog The Low Histamine Chef

Addendum – 2021

When I wrote this book, I stated in the first section that: "As far as I am aware, for most of us there is no cure for our salicylate/sulphur/amine/glutamate sensitivity and there is no quick fix." I would like to now revise that statement as I would say that I am cured and I can now freely eat whatever I want and go about my life with only the occasional mild salicylate sensitivity issue. How did it happen? – I learned to love myself and focus on what I felt good about.

How Letting Go Led to My Healing
Your physical and emotional body naturally align with the universal energy of love and wellbeing when you let go of resistance with your mind. You do not have to try to heal yourself. Simply focus on what you feel good about and do things you love. Fun, laughter, play and connecting to nature are the best paths to both emotional and physical healing.

I know this may sound simplistic, and possibly a little new-agey, but that is how my healing happened. I had immersed myself in trying to learn about human health and with finding out how to cure myself. Then one day, I realised that all my research was actually creating stress and fear in me as I was overanalysing everything. I was tying myself up in knots in my head from all the information that I was focusing on. Then I had this "aha" moment that I did not need to be well (fixed) to be happy, as in I did not need to put my life on hold until I was better and healed. I decided to stop focusing on getting well, and to start focusing on being happy.

I gathered up all my health books and gave them away and

decided to simply focus on feeling good in whatever way I could. It was from this that I launched my website The Feel Good Life Club (this has since evolved into my current website, janinelattimore.com), and began the practices which I outline in my book *10 Steps to Happiness*. I began to focus on tuning into my own intuition and my body's wisdom, rather than doing too much external research.

It is a common human tendency to want to fix whatever is wrong rather than focus on what is going well and what we like. It is an expression of the human negativity bias I think; a learned survival behaviour which is based in fear.

Healing Happens from the Heart
The concept I am talking about here is not one of false positivity where you avoid dealing with issues, hurts or uncomfortable emotions. Rather, I am talking about shifting your mindset to one of acceptance and love. It is a shift from trying to understand and fix things in your head, to letting them heal from your heart. This is in line with the research of Dr Joe Dispenza, Bruce Lipton and the HeartMath Institute, and the teachings of people such as Katherine Woodward Thomas, and Gay Hendricks and the collective consciousness that is called Abraham Hicks.

"Because our heart is emanating a coherent field when we open it, we start feeling less polarized, less analytical, and less anxious. The result is that we begin to see life through a different prism. That frequency generated from elevated emotions carries information, so as an example, when a person changes their energy and starts laying down the thought of health or wealth, that thought of health or wealth can be carried on that frequency. The thought of health can't be carried on the frequency or emotion of suffering because they are different frequencies, thus they carry a different set of thoughts and information.

. . . if your energy is high enough, then your energy can literally entrain someone else to an elevated frequency. We now see this regularly when we do coherence healings at our workshops, resulting in instantaneous, miraculous changes from blindness to perfect sight, deafness to hearing, tumors disappearing, stage-4 cancer going into remission, Parkinson's Disease, MS and Lupus disease reversing, shifts in kidney functions (such as kidney failure), changes in the brain, and so on and so on."
- Dr Joe Dispenza – Heal Yourself, Heal Others Part 1 and 2

The Healing Power of Self-Acceptance
The first book I read when I began this stage of my healing journey was Louise Hay's book *You Can Heal Your Life*. While I think this book has much to offer, the concept of repeating affirmations hundreds of times a day felt overwhelming to me at that point in my life. The next book I read was Gay Hendrick's book *Learning to Love Yourself*. The process he describes for loving yourself for whatever you are feeling is so simple, but has been, and still is, one of the most healing practices I engage in. I describe how to do my version of it in my book *10 Steps to Happiness*.

So where does this leave you having just bought this book?
Healing usually takes time. If you are in the midst of stress in dealing with chemical sensitivity issues, then the practical information in this book will help you to manage and reduce your symptoms. Remember, this is where I started, so it is not a waste to have bought this book. However, I recommend that once you feel like you are managing your symptoms effectively and want to move into further healing then also get my book *10 Steps to Happiness* and start working your way through the information and practices in it. This will help you move into healing on an emotional and energetic level.

Introduction

How This Book Can Help You – Please read this first
There are some good books and resources available about what causes food intolerances, how to identify them, elimination diet protocols, food lists and recipe ideas. What I struggled to find was a book on how to get better. I didn't want myself and my children to have to live on severely restricted diets, and I didn't want to live my life in constant anxiety that I would inhale, touch or consume something that would cause my skin to erupt in painful, ugly spots, rashes and itching. To avoid all the things we reacted to we would have to live in a bubble surviving on a diet of lettuce, celery, boiled fresh meat, rice, pears and banana. I found information about treatments and remedies scattered across forums and blogs, but no book that put it all together in a practical way. So, I wrote one.

Free to Eat outlines what I have found out by research and then trial and error to reduce the food intolerance symptoms caused by histamine, sulphur, glutamate and salicylate sensitivity in myself and my children. It is the 'how to' handbook I wish someone had given me after we had identified our food intolerances and chemical sensitivities. While I read scientifically researched information to identify treatments, this book simply outlines the remedies themselves that we, and fellow chemical intolerance sufferers, find effective. There are very few 'why' explanations, just the 'what to do' based on what experience has shown to be effective. I wanted to keep this book as basic to read as possible, because I myself found that some of the information available about these intolerances is very technical and sometimes all I wanted was a basic explanation of what I could do to manage our illness. *Free to Eat* is an easy-to-follow step by step plan to reducing your food intolerance reactions so that you can eat a wide variety of foods and live a relatively normal life.

Free to Eat will help you reduce the symptoms of your chemical intolerance and increase your tolerance levels by showing you how to:

- Implement quick easy strategies to reduce stress
- Incorporate enjoyable exercise into your life
- Eat and drink the right things in the right way to heal your body
- Groom yourself to look good using chemical-free/safe products (including make-up, hair-styling and hair removal)
- Use safe treatments for day-to-day ailments (including reducing cold symptoms, easing itching, and reducing reaction symptoms quickly)
- Take minimal effective nutritional supplements to boost your body's digestive and detoxification function
- Keep your home hygienically clean using chemical-free/safe products

And much more.

I am sharing this information simply because this is what works for us, and because I want to help other people with chemical intolerances as I know how difficult they can make our lives.

This book is written for people who have already identified that they have an intolerance or sensitivity to one or more of the following: salicylates, histamines/amines, sulphur and glutamates. It may seem ambitious or even a little confusing to write a book covering all these chemical intolerances, but the reason I have is because it is quite common that if you suffer from one chemical intolerance, you also experience intolerance to other chemicals (I suffer from them all). Moreover, many of the management strategies in terms of lifestyle and supplementation are the same for all of these chemical sensitivities.

Free to Eat does not cover the symptoms of chemical/food intolerance, how to identify which chemicals you are sensitive to or elimination diet protocols. It also does not include food lists because it covers so many different chemicals and this is well covered in other resources. For information regarding symptoms, identification, elimination diets and food lists see the resources listed in the appendix at the end of this book.

I send you much love as I know the challenges of this journey, but healing and full recovery are possible.

Disclaimer
Throughout this publication statements are made pertaining to the properties and/or function of food and/or nutritional products. While every effort has been made to provide accurate information, these statements are not intended to diagnose, treat, cure or prevent any disease. Please seek the advice of a qualified health professional before implementing significant changes to your diet or taking health supplements. If you are taking prescription medication, then consult a qualified health professional before making changes to the medication you are taking. Janine Lattimore is not responsible for any actions taken on the basis of information contained within this publication nor for any error of omission contained herein. Janine Lattimore disclaims all liability in respect of anything done or not done in reliance upon all or part of the contents of this publication.

Contents

The Fourfold Aim	15
Step 1: The First Step to Getting Better	23
Parasites and infections	24
Allergies	27
Eliminate Environmental Chemicals First	27
Step 2 – Live A Healing Lifestyle	29
Manage Stress Effectively	29
Enjoy Exercise	42
Sleep	45
Stay Hydrated	46
Keep Cool	48
Have Pampering Showers	49
Venturing Out and About	50
How to Manage Social Situations	50
Managing Partners/Spouses	53
Step 3 - Eat the Right Things in the Right Way	59
Avoid The Inflammatory 5	60
Eat Adequate Protein	72
Prioritise Nutrition	75
Eat Organic where possible	82
Chew Your Food Thoroughly	83
Eat Adequate Amounts	83
Keep Your Salt Intake Low	85
Eat The Right Fats	86
Reintroducing Foods	89
Rotating Foods	90
Desensitisation	90

Step 4: Avoid Chemicals (Without Avoiding Life) — 103
Personal Care — 104
Food Handling and Storage — 118
Cleaning — 122
Clearing the Air — 124
Treating Day to Day Illness — 125
Odd Extras — 131

Step 5: Add Effective Supplements — 135
The Core Supplements — 140
Sulphate, magnesium and zinc — 140
Probiotics — 144
Vitamin D — 151
Digestive Enzymes — 152
Vitamin K — 156
Biotin — 157
Iron — 158
Molybdenum — 159
Selenium — 159
Vitamin B12 — 160
L-Histidine — 161
Omega 3 — 162
Calcium — 163

Appendices — 165
EFT for Food Intolerances — 165
Resources — 170

The Fourfold Aim

Free to Eat outlines numerous measures that you can take in terms of personal care, cleaning, leisure, lifestyle and nutritional supplementation to help you reduce your chemical sensitivities. The measures discussed in this book are based around a fourfold aim:

The Fourfold Aim:
1. Heal your digestive system and improve its functioning
2. Calm and strengthen your immune system
3. Reduce inflammation in your body
4. Increase the efficiency of your body's detoxification pathways

Between my two children and I, we experience intolerance and sensitivities to: salicylates, amines/histamine, sulphur, glutamates, gluten, eggs, soy, corn, fructose, citric acid and dairy. These intolerances/sensitivities were identified through many months (years) of following an elimination diet and keeping daily food diaries coupled with visits to a dietician who specialized in chemical intolerances. Our main symptoms and specific intolerances differ slightly, but we share most of the above in common. I mainly experience symptoms in my skin such as hives, eczema and acne, but I also experience brain fog, intense anxiety, fatigue, excessive hunger, back pain, muscle pain, very low blood pressure and low blood sugar levels. My daughter mainly exhibits behavioural symptoms such as making constant nonsense sounds, being excessively defiant/contrary, excessive emotional responses/tantrums, overly loud talking and difficulty going to sleep and staying asleep. She also experiences brain fog, anxiety, increased hunger (we call it 'the hungries') and excessive forgetfulness (e.g., she will ask the same question repeatedly over a short space of time forgetting she has asked it or what the answer was). My son mainly experiences gut pain and discomfort, but also excessive agitation/mild hyperactivity at times. When I wrote this book, my son had just turned four and as he was so young and had experienced issues with most foods it was difficult to tell if he had the same chemical sensitivities as my daughter and I or rather an extremely sensitive gut. As he has gotten older, I have been able to clarify that he does actually have many of the same chemical sensitivity issues, though his salicylate sensitivity is milder than mine and my daughter's, but his citric acid intolerance was much higher.

At first, I tried just avoiding food and environmental triggers as much as possible. However, with our extensive list of intolerances this was very hard to manage and I began to feel uncomfortable restricting my children's diet so much. I was also struggling to get enough to eat and had lost so much weight that I looked like I had an eating disorder. It was almost impossible to avoid exposure to environmental triggers such as the cleaning products used at school and kindergarten, and friends and family members' perfumes/body sprays etc. My research indicated that the problem we had was a genetic issue and if you had it then you had it for life. Although I have only recently found out about these chemical intolerances and identified the symptoms in myself, observing my daughter's symptoms and thinking back to my own behaviour as a child leads me to believe that I have had these chemical sensitivities all my life, though never as severely as I currently have them. Thus, I didn't think that I or my daughter would 'grow out' of these intolerances and that instead I needed to find a way to reduce our reactions as much as possible.

I began a long period of research and experimentation to try and identify what helped us reduce our symptoms and increase our food and chemical intolerance levels. I then organised the information I gained into the plan that is outlined in this book. Following the steps in this plan has helped my children and I to manage our intolerances effectively and live relatively normal lives. My hope in sharing this information is that it will help others find a way to successfully manage and reduce their chemical intolerance symptoms faster and with less work and stress than I experienced.

The Free to Eat plan is divided into steps. The reason for this is because depending on your level of intolerance and individual biological make-up, you may not need to complete the whole plan in order to manage or even eliminate your intolerances. Some people may only need to manage their stress levels effectively and get more exercise and sleep in order to reduce their intolerance symptoms. Other people, like myself, may need to implement every step outlined in the plan. The steps start from basic changes to your lifestyle and environment and progress through to a range of core supplements that can help your body detoxify chemicals more effectively and heal your digestive and immune system. Start with Step 1 and progress through each of the following steps in turn until you are experiencing a significant improvement in your tolerance levels and reduction in your symptoms.

As far as I am aware, for most of us there is no cure for our salicylate/sulphur/amine/glutamate sensitivity and there is no quick fix. I have heard of some cases where children have been 'cured', but I am sceptical as to whether they have been completely healed or whether their tolerance levels are just currently very high, or possibly even that they actually had a sensitive gut which they have just grown out of. I have not read of any adults with chemical sensitivities being 'cured'.

What I have observed in myself, my children and others is that you can reduce the symptoms of your reactions by various means, and you can increase your tolerance levels, but the condition itself never fully goes away and tends to just get better when your body is stronger and worse when it is challenged by diet and/or stress. Thus, although it might be tempting to skip to the nutritional supplement section of this book in the hopes that you can just take a 'pill' and all will be well, unfortunately that is not the case. Our bodies are far too complex and too many different factors impact on our health for a 'pill' to effectively manage a systemic (whole body) issue like chemical intolerance.

Reducing your reactions and healing your body takes time and a commitment to caring for yourself body and soul. That is why step one of the Free to Eat plan is all about choosing to live a lifestyle that nurtures your physical, emotional and mental health. Your emotional and mental health has been scientifically shown to have a significant effect on your physical health. Healing requires learning to love your body and treat it with the respect and care it needs.

Do I have to give up everything?
Does this mean you have to avoid everything for the rest of your life? Firstly, we can't live in the modern world without being exposed to chemicals. They infuse the air we breathe, the people we interact with and the buildings we live in and use. As we are exposed to so many chemicals incidentally in ways beyond our control we need to try and reduce as much chemical exposure in things that we do have control over as we can. In terms of food, I am careful with my diet when I am preparing the food, and if I'm going to a pot-luck type meal then I take something suitable for myself and my children. If I am going out to a cafe/restaurant or to someone's house where they have prepared the meal then I try to avoid anything very high in the chemicals I react to, but relax about

everything else and just enjoy the food as a treat. There is an anti-smoking campaign advertisement that used to on here in New Zealand that stated "every cigarette is doing you damage". The same is true for those of us with chemical intolerances. Every time we are exposed to a chemical we react to, it causes damaging inflammation in our bodies and this damage accumulates over time with repeated exposures. In light of this I try to limit my exposure as much as I can when I can so that it is alright when I occasionally experience exposure when I cannot avoid it. It is about balance – keeping your chemical levels low whenever it is practical so that the occasional high exposure doesn't cause too many issues.

You will need to change some of your habits and the way you look at things. Identify 'safe' treats for when you feel the need for something special or something comforting. You may not be able to have chocolate any more, but depending on your particular intolerances you may still be able to have white marshmallows or carob brownies or rice pudding when you feel like something sweet. Better still identify things that make you feel good that improve your health too like having a pamper weekend away or watching a movie or listening to some music you like or buying an article of clothing you really want. Instead of seeing it as missing out on things I see it as choosing to feel and look good. I choose to avoid the things I react to because I believe that the benefits of doing so are well worth it. You have the power to choose your perspective and choosing a positive one improves your mental and physical health and creates an attractive environment in your life. It did take me a while to fully come to this place of acceptance, but I am much happier now that I have.

A Note on Inflammation
Inflammation is part of your body's immune response to anything flagged as harmful or irritating. It is designed to be helpful. If you cut your arm, it is your body's inflammatory

response that will help your tissues heal and repair. Unfortunately, in our modern lifestyle our bodies are constantly flooded with inflammatory triggers. This causes chronic (on-going) low-grade inflammation which means there is a continuous presence of inflammatory chemicals circulating around your body and this can cause damage. When your immune system is constantly activated and inflammatory chemicals are constantly circulating, they are likely to start attacking harmless substances like food particles, beneficial bacteria and your own tissue cells. This is the cause of most modern disease and a major factor in chemical and food intolerances. When you continue to be exposed to foods and chemicals you are intolerant of it creates ongoing inflammation throughout your whole body including your brain. Conversely, the continuous presence of inflammatory chemicals in your gut - where 70% of your immune cells reside - can damage your intestinal barrier and lead to leaky gut, which is a common cause of food and chemical intolerance.

Inflammation affects your body and your brain. There is a direct physical connection in your body between your digestive system and your brain - it is called the gut brain axis. The microbiota in your gut, i.e., micro-organisms such as probiotic (good) bacteria, communicate with your central nervous system through neural, immune and hormonal pathways. This influences the function and behaviour of your brain. There is scientific evidence that your gut microbiota is involved in the regulation of pain, cognition, mood and anxiety. Chronic low-grade inflammation in your body can also make your blood-brain barrier leaky. This weakens your body's control over what enters your brain and can allow compounds to cross the blood-brain barrier that would normally be prevented from entering your brain.

Some common inflammatory triggers include:
- Bad (pathogenic) bacteria in our food, water and air, or bacterial or parasite infections in our body (the latter are more common than people realise)
- Environmental toxins (pesticides, PCBs, dioxins, xenoestrogens)
- Non-food based allergens (dust mites, pollen, dander)
- Inflammatory foods (refined sugars, refined vegetable oils, gluten, processed foods with chemical additives)
- Stress

Many of the help strategies outlined in this book are focused on reducing inflammation. Reducing inflammation may not completely cure your chemical intolerances, especially if they are caused by genetic enzyme deficiencies, but it will reduce the severity of your symptoms and help increase your tolerance levels.

Step 1: The First Step to Getting Better

Clarifying the Problem
I noted at the beginning that this book was for people who already knew that they had chemical sensitivities so it may seem strange to have 'clarifying the problem' as step one. The reason I have included this step is because I think that it is important to have a clear diagnosis of your specific intolerances, preferably obtained under the supervision of a trained health professional (see the Fed Up website for a list of suitable health professionals). Be very careful about self-diagnosing. Your symptoms may be caused by another health condition or you may eliminate foods from your diet unnecessarily. There are also a number of elimination diets available on the internet which are not written by qualified health professionals that may give you inaccurate or confusing results. Lastly, it is important to clearly know what your intolerances are before you begin taking nutritional supplements that may mask them. You can either go and see a doctor and have a thorough medical examination first, although be aware that most doctors do not support the connection between health issues and food intolerance, or you can see a dietician and undergo an authorised elimination diet first. If strictly following the elimination diet does not resolve your health issues, then seek further medical advice. When I first became ill, one thing I struggled with was identifying what tests needed to be done to identify the cause of the symptoms I was experiencing and who to see to get the support I needed. Since then, I have found a German article online that gives a clear outline of possible causes of food

intolerance issues and what tests aid in diagnosis which you can access at:
https://www.ncbi.nlm.nih.gov/pmc/articles/PMC2695393/

Parasites and Infections

It isn't a pleasant thought, but parasite infection is very common and you may be completely unaware that you are affected by it. Parasite and bacterial infections can cause similar symptoms to food and chemical intolerance. An article by Dr Amy Myers lists the following possible symptoms for parasite infections:

- You have unexplained constipation, diarrhoea, gas, or other symptoms of IBS
- You travelled internationally and remember getting traveller's diarrhoea while abroad
- You have a history of food poisoning and your digestion has not been the same since.
- You have trouble falling asleep, or you wake up multiple times during the night.
- You get skin irritations or unexplained rashes, hives, rosacea or eczema.
- You grind your teeth in your sleep.
- You have pain or aching in your muscles or joints.
- You experience fatigue, exhaustion, depression, or frequent feelings of apathy.
- You never feel satisfied or full after your meals.
- You've been diagnosed with iron-deficiency anaemia.

"Trouble sleeping, skin irritations, mood changes, and muscle pain can all be caused by the toxins that parasites release into the bloodstream. These toxins often cause anxiety, which can manifest itself in different ways. For instance, waking up in the middle of the night or grinding your teeth in your sleep are signs that your body is experiencing anxiety while you rest. When these toxins interact with your neurotransmitters or blood cells, they can cause mood swings or skin irritation." - Dr Amy Myers - mindbodygreen.com

A member on the Salicylatesensitivity.com forum noted: *"In many cases the sals/phenols intolerance will dissipate if Lyme is diagnosed properly and treated properly. Long term treatment is necessary if a patient has exhibited symptoms for longer than a few months. Most MD's are not educated on Lyme and will turn patients away, leaving them to suffer. You will have to be your own advocate to ask for highly specialized Lyme testing since the conventional tests are highly inaccurate. Go to www.ilads.org for info or friend the California Lyme Disease Association on Facebook for more information."*

Any form of infection in the body will also stimulate your immune system and increase inflammation which will lower your tolerance levels and increase the incidence and severity of symptoms. The most common treatments for parasites and bacterial infections are antibiotics or herbal remedies, both of which are likely to cause issues for those of us with chemical intolerances, but sometimes it can be beneficial to bear with it for the course of the treatment in order to clear the infection. Antibiotic medication may be better tolerated if it is prepared by a compounding pharmacist who can prepare a formulation free from additives and colouring.

Personally, I tried using a frequency generator, commonly called a Zapper, which is a device that "electrocutes" small pathogens such as parasites, bacteria, viruses, fungus and other toxins. I am aware that there is significant controversy about the science behind these devices and the effectiveness of them, but my experience was very positive. I used, and still regularly use, The Ultimate Zapper. When I started using it, I was very ill. I was suffering from chronic fatigue and had just started seeing a counsellor for significant anxiety and depression. I had multiple chemical sensitivity and my tolerance levels were extremely low.

Within the first few weeks of using the frequency generator I experienced significant flu-like symptoms, but my energy levels began to increase. The most startling thing I noticed was that my anxiety just seemed to disappear – it was like someone had lifted a dark, smothering blanket off me. I began to go about my day smiling to myself simply because I felt good for no apparent reason. A few weeks into treatment I happened to give myself an Epsom salt footbath right after using the frequency generator and when I went to tip the water out of the bowl, I noticed several worm-like threads in the water. I had never noticed anything like that before when I had given myself a footbath treatment and it was not fluff. I am sure they were worm casings which had been drawn out by the footbath. A few days later when I repeated this procedure there was a bug-like casing left in the footbath water. It was not like a bug had gotten into the water, it looked like a parasite casing.

Based on this experience it appears that I had a parasite infection consisting of several different parasites, and that the frequency generator I used killed most if not all of these. The flu-like symptoms faded after the first 4-5 weeks of treatment and my anxiety did not return. My energy levels returned to normal. I felt physically and mentally like a great weight had been lifted from me. After I had been using the frequency generator for 2-3 months my histamine, sulphur and citric acid intolerances began to decrease significantly and are now minimal if not gone. I have also been using the device with my children and have noticed that their histamine, sulphur and citric acid intolerances are now also minimal if not gone. My salicylate and glutamate intolerances have reduced slightly, but are still quite high however, and it is the same with my children.

The frequency generator I use plugs into the wall. If you have safety concerns about using a device that plugs into the mains electricity you can get battery operated frequency generators.

Test for Allergies Before Altering Your Diet
If you have not yet changed your diet, then I would recommend being tested for allergies before starting an elimination diet. It is wise to ascertain whether allergies are a problem and this can only be tested in some ways while you are still consuming substances that you are allergic too. When your body is exposed to things it is allergic to it increases histamine and inflammation in your body. Get a medical blood allergy test performed for such things as gluten, dairy, sugar, corn, soy, nuts and eggs etc. However, be aware that blood allergy tests are not 100% accurate and do not identify intolerances. It is a good starting point though to gain further insight into your health issues before you begin an elimination diet.

Eliminate Environmental Chemicals Before Altering Your Diet
If you have not already eliminated high chemical foods from your diet, then I would recommend eliminating environmental sources of chemicals first. The reason I advise this is because for some people eliminating environmental sources of chemicals may be enough to significantly reduce or clear your symptoms. I do not advocate restricting your diet unless you have to, and cleaning and personal care products contribute greatly to total chemical intake.

Please note: for some people a sudden decrease in exposure to salicylates can cause increased salicylate sensitivity and/or detoxification issues including a worsening of symptoms such as hives/eczema/itching, digestive disturbance, head or body aches or cold-like symptoms for example a runny nose. I don't think this causes any harm, but it can be uncomfortable and confusing. For this reason, you may wish to reduce your, or your child's, exposure slowly to reduce the severity of any response.

I am aware that clearly identifying food and chemical intolerances can be a long and often frustrating process, and that most of us just want to get better as fast as possible. It took me two to three years to fully identify my own and my children's food and chemical intolerances and it was a trying time for all of us, but it is important to go through this process to gain an understanding of your personal health issues. You need this knowledge as a basis to work from.

I also recommend working with a qualified health professional. I know that this can be costly, but think of it as an investment. Food and chemical intolerances are a contributing factor to many other health issues such as arthritis, asthma, Crohn's disease, migraines, sexual dysfunction and tinnitus. For this reason, identifying and managing them is a worthwhile investment in your long term health, comfort and enjoyment of life. An understanding health professional can also provide valuable support. Except for those relating to gluten, dairy and egg, most other food and chemical intolerances are not widely accepted by the general population yet, and I found that many people thought it was all in my head, or just didn't understand and so didn't know how to support me.

Step 2 – Live A Healing Lifestyle

Manage Stress Effectively
Stress is probably the number one factor in modern day ill health. I recommend that it is the primary thing for you to focus on managing, which is why I have made it the first 'treatment' discussed in this book. Reducing stress in your life can be enough on its own to produce significant improvements in your health and, conversely, failing to do so can decrease the effectiveness of other treatments to the point of making them a waste of time. All my research has brought me back to this: effective stress management is key. Make it your ongoing top priority to keep your stress levels low. Invest the majority of your time, effort and financial outlay in this because it will give you the best results.

Make sure you have someone appropriate to 'unload' to, whether it be a professional counsellor or a friend; find a way to forgive and let go of hurts and grudges; heal or remove yourself from difficult relationships; attend classes in yoga, Qigong, Tai Chi and meditation; find something you enjoy and do it daily; have fun. These are the best things you can do to reduce the symptoms of your chemical sensitivities and improve your tolerance levels.

Choose to accept that it is okay to let go, go slow, unplug, nap and do things just for pleasure. The modern world is so full of opportunities that we fear we will miss out if we are not constantly plugged in, but we are missing out on pleasuring our own soul. Try to simplify your life and home as much as possible and remove yourself from the constant barrage of marketing, distraction and noise. Instead of watching TV or some other digital device in the evening try sitting in the moonlight and doing something creative like playing a musical instrument or drawing. Even if you start with having just one technology free evening a week it is a positive step, and making changes one step at a time is the best way to establish ongoing habits.

How Stress Affects You
When you are stressed, your digestive system works less effectively and you are prone to higher levels of inflammation. Prolonged physical, emotional or psychological stress can:
- cause hormonal imbalances
- raise blood sugar levels which stimulates the release of more insulin. High insulin levels promote inflammation throughout your body and brain.
- decrease beneficial gut flora populations, which can weaken your immune function
- stimulate the overgrowth of yeast and pathogenic (bad) bacteria in your gut
- cause harmful bacteria to cling to your intestinal tract causing damage
- decrease enzymatic output in your gut by as much as 20,000-fold
- trigger or heighten food and chemical sensitivities
- cause mast cells to release histamine which can cause or worsen allergic symptoms
- decrease the flow of oxygen in your blood and to your brain promoting inflammation in your brain
- cause the excretion of nutrients, such as water-soluble vitamins and calcium

Even smaller episodes of stress, such as when you have a cold, cause your immune system to work extra hard which can result in your chemical tolerance levels decreasing for a time.

An angry argument can stimulate a chemical sympathetic stress response in your body that lasts for several days.

Do something every day that you find enjoyable and relaxing even if it is just sitting down for 15 minutes with your feet up to read a book. Be aware of not taking on too much. Learn to say 'no' if you do not want to, or feel you do not have the capacity to, do something. Respect your own needs. The world will not fall down if you do not do everything you feel you should or that other people want you to. Learn to delegate, especially to your children as it teaches them valuable life skills.

Strategies you can use to keep your stress levels down

Be realistic

Stress is often caused by the difference between our expectations and reality i.e., we expect that something will happen or someone will do something and then it doesn't happen or the person doesn't do what we thought. We can only change and manage ourselves. Often, we expect too much of ourselves, and others, and life. I find that the following Serenity Prayer is great wisdom to try and live by:

> *Grant me the serenity to accept the things I cannot change,*
> *the courage to change the things I can,*
> *and the wisdom to know the difference.*

Learn to let go of unrealistic expectations of yourself and others. Set just one goal for yourself each day. If someone constantly fails to do what you want, then think about why that might be. Are you expecting something from them that is out of character or impractical? Do you need to voice your desire clearly to them i.e., have you even told them what you want? Women especially tend to have the expectation that if our partners loved us, they would just know what we wanted, and then we get disappointed when they don't give us what we want. Nobody is a mind reader and generally men are not very intuitive about the feelings and desires of others. We do not live in a romance novel. Learn to effectively communicate what you want.

We also need to be realistic about our chemical intolerances. Most of us get intimately attuned to every subtle change in our bodies. 'Regular' people tend not to constantly examine every change in their body like we do. It is very easy to become obsessive. Accept that you will probably always have symptoms to some degree. Let go of the expectation of being perfectly cured, unfortunately it is not realistic and will cause you to feel frustration and despair. Envision yourself getting better, because positive thinking is healing, but hold the vision lightly with love and let go of striving for perfection.

Breathe, Smile and be Thankful

I view these as my core 'get happy' helpers. They are all quick and easy to do, can be done anywhere by anyone with no equipment necessary, and they produce significant results. When you breathe deeply you expand and contract your diaphragm. This stimulates your lymphatic system and massages your internal organs. Your lymphatic system removes excess fluid, waste and toxins from your body's cells and tissues and works with your circulatory system to deliver nutrients and oxygen from your blood to your cells. Deep breathing from your abdomen/diaphragm also switches off your body's sympathetic nervous system stress response and switches on your relaxation oriented parasympathetic nervous system. Lastly, deep breathing helps to reduce inflammation in your body. I think it is amazing that something so simple and enjoyable can help us relax, energise, fuel-up and detox. Learn to breathe properly (I have outlined a simple exercise below to help you with this) and whenever you feel stressed take a few moments to breathe deeply. When you are waiting in line or in the car use the time to breathe deeply, or make it your daily hit of happiness (see below) by taking ten minutes to sit, or lie on your back, and breathe (if the weather permits, you can lie on the grass and imagine cloud pictures at the same time).

The physical act of smiling, whether or not we feel the emotions behind it, can elicit the same response in our body as genuine smiling. Of course, it is good to build things into your life that make your smile with joy as well, but even just physically adjusting the muscles on your face into a grin has benefits (it also exercises the muscles on your face helping to keep your facial muscles toned). Smiling stimulates the release of feel-good serotonin and endorphins, reduces stress and strengthens your immune system. It also helps us to maintain a positive mindset as it is hard to focus on something negative when you are smiling. Smiling also makes you look younger and more attractive. Get a little Mona Lisa style and cultivate a habitual mysterious smile.

Focusing on things that you are thankful for can quickly reduce stress and worry. You could try this simple exercise: before you go to sleep think of, or write down in a journal, at least 5 things that you are thankful for right now. They do not need to be big - it could be just that you are happy to have a warm bed, or that your cat gave you a cuddle. Think back over the day that has been and interpret it in terms of things to be thankful for instead of mistakes made or things left undone. I find this helps me to sleep more restfully. I also turn my mental focus to things to be thankful for when I am starting to feel overwhelmed by things to do, or by worry.

Quick Tip: A fast easy relaxation activity you can do before bed, or first thing in the morning or anytime you need a stress break is to sit somewhere quiet, breathe fully into your abdomen, physically smile and think of things you are thankful for (you can simply be thankful that you are able to breathe, that you are breathing and alive, that your body is relaxing, that you can smile, that you are able to feel good, that you are allowed to feel good or that it is okay to take time for you). Even 5 minutes of this makes a big difference to your wellbeing.

Abdomen Breathing Exercise
Do this exercise somewhere quiet where you won't be disturbed for 10-15 minutes. Lie on your back on the floor. Ensure you are comfortable, put a cushion under your head if you want, but it is best to lie on a firm, flat surface (avoid lying on a bed as you will likely fall asleep). Let your feet fall out naturally and place your arms by your sides a little out from your body with your palms up. There is no exact position and the key is to adjust yourself so that you are comfortable. This pose is known as Corpse Pose in yoga and is very relaxing. Close your eyes. Let your face relax and your body sink into the floor.

Next, place one hand on your chest and one hand on your abdomen (belly button). Take a slow deep breath in through your nose. Nose breathing correlates with your relaxation response and parasympathetic nervous system. The object of this exercise is to breathe into the hand on your abdomen first and 'fill-up' your body with the hand on the chest rising last. Pause, then exhale by pouring the air out of your chest first then down to your abdomen last. Your belly is the powerhouse. Draw the air in from your abdomen and push it out from there. You might like to imagine that your abdomen is like a set of bellows drawing air in and pushing it out. Alternatively, you can imagine the process as being like filling a jug with water, filling the bottom first then rising to the top and then emptying it from the top all the way to the last drop at the bottom. Think about your breathing, but try to let it flow as naturally as possible. Avoid forcing anything and if you get out of pattern just take a normal breath and then begin again. There is no right or wrong, just practice and growth. This time is just for you. No one else is judging you so let go of any judgements of yourself.

Breathe this way for 5-15 minutes (or more if you want) until you feel deeply relaxed. When you get up, roll onto your side first and get up slowly as you may feel a little light headed. This is just one of many possible deep breathing exercises, but it is a good one to start with as it is so simple. There are many more options detailed on the internet.

Relax to Eat
It can help reduce food intolerance reactions simply by sitting down, breathing deeply and taking your time when you eat. Avoid eating when you are feeling stressed, angry or upset and take some time to calm down first. Sitting down and taking three full, slow abdominal breaths before you eat is usually all you need to start to relax. You also digest food more effectively if you eat away from the TV, tablet/iPad or any other stimulating device or environment. Avoid watching/reading the news when you are eating because it is often negative. Reading a light, enjoyable fiction book is okay, but it is best to just engage in light conversation while you eat or use the opportunity to just be in the moment, or gaze out a window and daydream. If you are at work, take your lunch-break and get away from your work area to sit and eat lunch. If you can, it is also very beneficial to go for a brisk walk outside either before or after you eat, even if it is only for 10 minutes. The exercise will help you to de-stress, enable your digestive system to work better, and boost your energy levels for the afternoon helping to prevent mid-afternoon sugar cravings.

I have recently come back to doing nothing when I eat apart

from sitting, eating and calmly engaging with others when they are present. I used to do this and then I started using the time when I was eating to read. While reading can be relaxing, I was reading to use, i.e., not waste, that time. For me reading while eating was a way of multi-tasking. As I have come back to doing nothing while I eat, I have noticed some things. Firstly, I chew my food more and eat more slowly. Secondly, I feel calm and relaxed after my meal whereas I used to often feel stimulated or annoyed. When I tried to read while eating my children would often interrupt my reading and I would get frustrated that I couldn't even have ten minutes peace to sit and read my book. Now, I don't mind when my children talk to me while I am eating and I often just sit and watch and listen to them. I have also noticed that not only do I feel more relaxed, but the calm seems to flow to them and my husband. My relationship with my children has improved. My daughter has picked up my habit of reading when she eats. It is better than watching a digital device, but now looking at her I see how it shuts out the people around you and I presume that my children, and husband, felt that when I was reading.

At first, I struggled with 'doing nothing' while I ate and I found that listening to slower, soulful music helped me transition. It gave me a focus. Now I am happy just sitting enjoying the feel of the food in my mouth, listening, watching, reflecting, dreaming (visualising), breathing and indulging in a period of mental space. I also find that I do not feel as fatigued as I used to.

If you have children, then try and make mealtimes enjoyable and relaxing. As often as possible turn off digital devices and sit together to have meals. Listen to music, chat or play word games like Twenty Questions (Animal, Mineral, Vegetable), Two Truths and One Lie, Would You Rather? or tell a made-up story with each person in turn adding a sentence or two.

Use open ended questions to stimulate conversation such as "What was the funniest thing you heard all day?"; "did someone do something nice for you today?"; "what was the hardest thing you had to do today?", or "what is the thing you are looking forward to most tomorrow?" Sometimes asking an unexpected question attracts more of your child's attention, for example "if you could fly for free anywhere in the world where would you go and why?"

Get Your Daily Happiness Hit:
Find a way to relax that works for you and practice it daily - make it your daily hit of happy. This could be:
- Going for a walk (especially in natural surroundings)
- Practicing yoga/Qigong/Tai chi
- Singing (join a local choir or put on your favourite music and sing without worrying if you sound any good)
- Swimming
- Playing with a pet
- Doing something creative, even just colouring-in
- Reading an entertaining book

Remember the Sabbath
In the Christian bible God gives everyone the right to have one day off a week – the Sabbath. Traditionally this is a Sunday and a day to focus on spiritual things. Your day off doesn't have to be a Sunday, but it is very beneficial to book in one day off each week. For those of us Type A personalities who find it hard to stop - you can do it, just let go and remember that it is your God-given right to have it. If you find it too much to take a whole day off at least take half.

Diary in your day off first. Make it a priority not a leftover or something you'll squeeze in if you have time after everything else is done. Leave other things undone. This is important. You are important and so is your health. You also don't have to go to church, but it would be a good idea to invest some time in some sort of soul enriching activity. For some this may be meditating, for others watching a movie, for others going surfing, or for others creating a work of art or craft. Soul enriching activities are those that we enjoy and feel refuelled emotionally after engaging in. What do you consistently want to do 'when you have the time'? What did you enjoy doing when you were a child?

Learn to Communicate Effectively
Learning how to ask clearly for what you need and to deal with conflict in a calm pro-active manner is very important in helping to manage sources of stress in relationships. Attend workshops, listen to web talks or read books about how to communicate effectively with your partner, family and children. It is a very worthwhile investment of your time.

Helping Kids Relax
Fortunately, kids have a naturally affinity for fun and laughter if left to their own devices and the best way to help your children relax is to slow down and relax yourself. Some children are more prone to anxiety than others, though I found my children's anxiety levels drop considerably when I can keep their chemical exposure low. Here are a few tips for helping your children avoid excess stress:

- **allow them enough down-time**: avoid enrolling children in too many activities/classes like sports, music, dance etc. One or two extra activities on top of pre-school/school is usually enough. Some children are fine doing a lot of extra activities and some struggle with just one. Listen to your child. Constructive play is just as beneficial to their development as music lessons.

- **establish effective bedtime routines**: help your children get plenty of sleep by having the same bedtime routine and bedtime every night except for special occasions. It is a good idea to have no technology (T.V., computer, electronic games etc.) for an hour before bed and include some wind-down activities like a bath/shower and/or reading stories together. My children also like a routine way of saying good-night. It could be a chat question like 'what did you like best about today' (teaching thankfulness), or a set good-night phrase like 'love you to the moon and back'.

- **have fun with them**: let your hair down and get crazy with your kids every so often - dance to a favourite song, play dress-ups, jump into their Xbox Kinect game, have a face-pulling competition or a tickle fight etc

- **teach your kids to breathe fully and correctly from the abdomen**

- **listen**: whenever your children talk do your best to pay attention and listen. When they are little, they may seem to go on (and on, and on) about little things, but if you develop your listening relationship with them when they are young, they are more likely to talk to you about more important things that are stressing them when they are older. Do your best to simply listen, paraphrase what they are saying and ask questions to help them see possible solutions for themselves. Avoid jumping in, lecturing or solving all their problems.

Stress Trauma

There is a physical connection between stress trauma and chemical sensitivities. While there are digestive aspects to some chemical sensitivities such as inefficient production or functioning of certain enzymes, for many of us with severe and multiple chemical sensitivities there is a neurological component as well. The neurological component is initiated by the amygdala area of the brain in response to an extremely stressful or traumatic event, and this event may be physical (e.g. breaking a bone or a parasite infection) or psychological. Ashok Gupta, Clinical Director of the Gupta Programme explains it this way:

During a particularly stressful period in someone's life, the amygdala is on high alert responding to emotional and physical threats. If the level of alert of the amygdala is particularly high, and the person is exposed to a toxin at the same time, a conditioned trauma can occur in the amygdala in association with the insula. . .
This conditioning occurs because when the amygdala is on high alert, it is very prone to learning new fears and sensitivities. Even if the original toxin did not present a threat to life, the amygdala will "err on the side of caution" in its hyper-anxious state, in order to protect the body.

From then on, any exposure to the original chemical, or any chemical which holds a vague resemblance to the original trigger, will initiate an over-stimulation of the sympathetic nervous system by the amygdala and hypothalamus, as well as specific reactions to mitigate the threat of the toxin. . .

The continuing over-stimulation of the sympathetic nervous system can cause secondary illnesses and issues, and is likely to suppress the effectiveness of the immune system.

The amygdala will also over-stimulate the brain, causing repetitive negative thoughts and feelings about the reactions, which themselves become hardwired into the brain. This reinforces the vicious cycles.

I did not identify my chemical sensitivities until I was in my forties and my symptoms became extreme. However, once I had identified them, I could recognise that I had experienced chemical sensitivities to a lesser degree for most of my life. Symptoms of my chemical sensitivities first became significant after I had a traumatic argument with my father when I was about age 10 or 11. My sensitivities became severe after I went through a period of high stress starting with the 2010-2011 series of earthquakes in Christchurch where I live, during which I also 'suffered' a late (I was 38), unplanned, difficult pregnancy. This was followed by the birth of my son who had acute digestive issues and hardly slept for two years. During this time my father had a stroke and my God-daughter, whom I am very close to, was being badly bullied and constantly running away from home. My children also experienced incidents of stress trauma via me while I was pregnant with them. My mother died of cancer when I was three months pregnant with my daughter, and I was about three months pregnant with my son when a violent earthquake struck Christchurch resulting in significant destruction and the death of 185 people.

Sometimes it is obvious when we have suffered a traumatic event. At other times the event is not so obvious or affects us more than we realise. I know I tend to suppress things. I don't like confrontation or getting overly emotional. I am calm in a crisis, but often that means that I do not fully process my feelings connected to it. Occasionally, we endure an event so traumatic that we mentally block it almost completely in order to cope.

If you suffer from severe chemical sensitivities and/or multiple chemical sensitivities, then I believe it is worthwhile seeking help to process any traumatic events that you have experienced, and to learn how to rewire your brain to correct negative patterns and fears concerning the substances you react to. Food intolerances can easily cause us to develop food phobias. I am aware that I now automatically think "I can't eat that" or feel a tightening grip of fear when I consider many foods, and that is an unhealthy food phobia.

There are several ways to address the psychological component of food and chemical sensitivities. Learning simple relaxation and meditation techniques are a good place to start. Being able to relax your mind and body when you begin to fear exposure to a particular toxin turns off your sympathetic nervous system stress response and increases your tolerance levels. This is also why it is very beneficial to sit, relax and do nothing else when you eat. I try to take a few full abdominal breaths before I begin eating a meal and repeat the following affirmations: deep breath – 'I am thankful for this food', deep breath – 'I choose to feel safe and relaxed when I eat', deep breath – 'all is well'/'everything is okay'.

You can take this a step further and learn some brain reprogramming techniques specifically for chemical sensitivities such as those taught by the Gupta Programme or the Dynamic Neural Retraining Programme (DNRP). If you want to seek help processing any traumatic experiences you have had then try and find a recommended therapist in your area. Therapists who are trained in hypnosis, Meridian Tapping/Emotional Freedom Technique or Neurolinguistic Programming (NLP) may also be able to assist you to release suppressed memories and emotions and retrain your brain. The most important thing with choosing a therapist is that it is someone you trust and feel comfortable being completely open with.

I personally used a Meridian Tapping technique to help let go of negative mental and emotional responses to food. I have written this out and included it in the appendix of this book.

Enjoy Exercise
If managing your stress levels effectively is the number one best thing you can do to reduce your chemical sensitivity symptoms and increase your tolerance levels, then exercising regularly is number two.
Here are some of the benefits of exercise:
- ➢ Regular moderate exercise strengthens your immune

- system and increases your tolerance levels.
- ➢ Exercise circulates lymph fluid around your body through the lymph vessels. Lymph circulates immune cells and carries waste out of your body.
- ➢ Exercise causes us to draw in more oxygen and circulates oxygen, nutrients and immune cells throughout your body via the bloodstream. Adequate supply of oxygen to your brain is necessary to keep it functioning well, and prevent brain inflammation.
- ➢ Exercise increases the efficiency of your bloodstream carrying waste products out of your body (i.e., exercise increases detoxification)
- ➢ Exercise stimulates the thymus gland and speeds up the healing of intestinal cell walls.
- ➢ Regular, moderate exercise reduces inflammation in your body and brain

As Case Adams notes in his book *Natural solutions for Food Allergies and Food Intolerances*: *"exercise is one of the best and cheapest therapies available to boost immunity and tolerance."*

I can clearly observe a lessoning in my food intolerance symptoms when I exercise regularly, however avoid strenuous exercise as it stresses your body. Moderation is best. Exercise to a level where your heart rate is gently accelerated and you need to breathe quite deeply for about 30 minutes, or an hour for gentler forms of exercise like yoga. Brisk walking, yoga, jumping on a trampoline, hiking, dancing and playing team sports are all good forms of exercise, or you can join a gym and do one of the various classes it offers. Swimming is great exercise if you have access to a suitable chemical-free pool, lake or ocean, but avoid swimming in chlorinated public pools as it is like immersing yourself in toxic soup. Personally, my main form of exercise is hula hooping. I have been doing it for about 2 years. I find it a very enjoyable way to exercise. I also find that when I spend at least 5-10 minutes waist hooping every day that I can eat oats and legumes without digestive and back pain. I think this is due to the massaging effect of the hula hoop around my abdominal area. When I miss hooping for a few days the digestive and back pain return.

Avoid getting overheated when you exercise especially if you have a histamine intolerance (see Keep Cool below). In warmer weather exercise in the mornings or evenings when it is cooler, or go for a walk or bike ride in a forest where it is almost completely shaded (exercising around trees helps boost oxygen intake and oxygen helps our detoxification systems work more effectively).

Yoga is a good choice of exercise because combines the benefits of exercise with the benefits of deep meditative breathing. When practiced regularly it can effectively reduce stress and inflammation. Many yoga poses such as abdominal twists, downward dog, forward folds, legs up the wall, child's pose, cat's pose and triangle pose also massage and stimulate your digestive system, liver and kidneys enhancing detoxification.

I try to prioritise having an exercise session in the morning because if I leave it until later in the day, I often find it gets crowded out by other things or I just get too tired. My aim is to do at least 30 minutes of concentrated exercise a day. Teaming up with a friend can also help keep you motivated. You can also establish a regular fun activity to do with the kids like a Sunday morning family soccer game or midweek dance-off using a camera-based video game where you physically do the dance moves.

Sleep

"When you neglect sleep or have poor quality sleep, this registers as a significant stressor to your body. It makes you immune compromised, chubby, forgetful and crazy."
Robb Wolf - *The Paleo Solution*

Lack of sleep, along with stress and chemical toxins, elevates your body's inflammatory immune response making it prone to respond more strongly to allergens and toxins. This means that unless we avoid the foods and chemicals we are intolerant to we can get stuck in a debilitating cycle where chemical sensitivities cause sleep disturbance and then the sleep disturbance increases our inflammatory response making us react to more substances with greater reaction symptoms.

Managing stress effectively and enjoying regular exercise should help you to sleep more soundly. Here are some other things you may wish to try to promote better sleep:

Go to bed around between 10-10:30pm every night: Apart from the occasional special occasion aim to go to bed at a regular time around 10 - 10:30pm. This is considered by most the optimum time to retire for sleep.

Establish a wind-down routine: have a routine that you go through to prepare for bed and do it every night (this is also advisable for children). For example, my routine is to turn on my bedside lamp (cue bedtime), go to the toilet, brush my teeth, wash my face, perform a pressure point facial massage, put on my pyjamas and then do three quick, relaxing yoga postures.

Switch off: to help with relaxing and getting plenty of good quality sleep it is a good idea to switch off from all electronics including TV's, computers, smartphones and electronic games

1-2 hours before getting ready for bed. These electronics actually stimulate the brain and commonly cause disturbed sleep, physical stress and fatigue even though we may not be aware of it.

Keep cool: optimal room temperature for sleep is slightly cool, between 16-17 degrees Celsius or 60 to 68 degrees Fahrenheit. Being too hot or too cold can cause disturbed sleep.

Make it dark: to sleep really well you need to sleep in a room with no light. Hang block out blinds or thick dark curtains on the windows, switch off all electrical appliances such as televisions at the wall so they don't have stand-by lights glowing (ideally have no television in your bedroom). Consider getting a clock with an unlit screen where you can push a button and a light illuminates the time. If you must have a clock with a lit display, make sure the light colour is red which is less disturbing than blue or green.

Make it nice: make your bedroom all about great sleep and a place you feel attracted to relax in. Get the most comfortable bed you can, it is a very worthwhile investment, and cover it with attractive natural fibre bedding that will breathe and help keep your temperature regulated. Clear the room of clutter and work-related items - this is your sleep sanctuary.

Stay Hydrated
Drink plenty of clean water. Here are some of the benefits of drinking plenty of fresh clean water:
> The mucosal membrane in your intestines is largely water. If it gets dehydrated it thins and becomes less effective.

> Water aids digestion and the absorption of nutrients

> Water flushes and replenishes the digestive tract and is

necessary for the proper elimination of waste

- Your immune system utilizes water to produce lymph fluid. Lymph fluid circulates immune cells throughout your body and flushes toxins out.

- Water speeds the removal of toxins from every organ and tissue system in your body

- Water increases the availability of oxygen to cells

- Increased levels of histamine are released during periods of dehydration

Most tap water is high in contaminants and chemicals. Water is a crucial element in our body's detoxification system so it is important that you consume plenty of it, and that it is as free as possible from toxins itself. You want the water you drink to relieve your body's toxic load not add to it. It is best to drink either quality water from glass bottles, or water you filter yourself. If you have a sulphur intolerance, then you may react to mineralised water (I did). There are a number of different water filters available. Each has different properties and will suit different needs so I am not going to discuss them all in this book. See the resources section in the Appendix for links to recommended sources of information about water filters and bottled water.

Aim to consume around 8 glasses of pure water (2 litres) a day if you are 13 or older and 5-8 glasses (1-2 litres) if you are a child. I say consume rather than drink because water can also be obtained from high liquid foods like soup and stews, and from high liquid raw fruits and vegetables. However, water from drinks such as tea and coffee or flavoured/sweetened waters do not count towards our necessary water intake. Obviously, you will need to drink more if it is hot, or you exercise/sweat frequently, and you will need to drink less if you eat a lot of water containing foods like soups, stews, raw vegetables etc. It is helpful to drink a glass of water as soon as you get up in the morning to rehydrate and flush out the digestive system and body. From then on drink water freely throughout the day, but avoid drinking significant amounts just before, during or just after a meal as it dilutes your stomach acid and can inhibit digestion.

Two good indicators of whether you are consuming enough water are thirst and urine. If you feel thirsty your body is already dehydrated, so try to consume sufficient water that you do not experience thirst. When you are consuming sufficient water, your urine should be light yellow to clear with little or no odour unless you are taking B vitamins or other medications which would alter the colour and smell of it, or you have been eating asparagus. If you are consuming plenty of water and not taking anything else that would affect your urine, but it is still bright yellow or strongly odorous, then talk to a health professional as it may indicate another health issue.

Be aware that consuming too much water can also be a problem so listen to your body and aim for the middle road of enough, but not too much.

Keep Cool
Excess heat stimulates your body to release histamine. This is especially relevant for those of us with a histamine intolerance, but is also relevant for others as histamine and inflammation go hand in hand and high levels of inflammation in your body make reactionary symptoms worse. Wear layers so you can easily dress down or up as temperature fluctuates. Avoid sunbathing or being outside in the sun too much. A little sun exposure is good to obtain vitamin D, but it is best gained without getting too hot. Also

avoid drinking very hot drinks or eating very hot foods. Allow hot drinks and cooked meals to cool a little before consuming.

Have Pampering Showers
It doesn't take much to make your daily shower a detoxifying, relaxing experience. Start by dry body brushing your entire body, or giving yourself a massage. You can dry massage your skin or use an oil/lotion that you can tolerate. This may sound time consuming, and it does take a bit to learn the technique, but once you know what to do it takes 5-10 minutes to give yourself an invigorating rub-down. Massaging your skin helps to stimulate your body's circulation and lymphatic detoxification systems. There are a number of different body brushing and self-massage techniques available, but the basic idea is simply to start at your feet and stroke upwards towards your heart, moving up your legs to your torso, up each arm, then stroking up your neck front and back and finishing with a scalp massage. See the Recommended Resources section in the Appendix for more information on dry body brushing and lymphatic drainage self-massage. Personally, I use an Enjo microfiber body cloth to dry brush my skin as my skin is very sensitive, and I find even soft bristled brushes too irritating. I also give myself an acupressure point or lymphatic drainage facial massage while applying my jojoba oil 'moisturiser' after washing my face in the evening.

After your massage have a warm shower - avoid hot showers and long showers as when your body gets hot it releases histamine (see "Keep Cool" above). Finish with a cool rinse to cool your body and stimulate your circulation, but don't have it too cold as extreme cold also stimulates the release of histamine.

You can also 'massage' yourself in the shower and exfoliate

your skin at the same time by washing yourself with a microfibre glove. I use an Enjo microfiber body glove and find it very effective. I can use it without any soap or body wash and find that it leaves my skin feeling very smooth. My skin has also been less dry since I started using microfibre cloths without cleansers to wash my face and body.

Venturing Out and About

The best leisure activities are those that involve activity outside among nature. Swimming pools, shopping malls and roadsides contain concentrations of chemicals and are best avoided. Going for a walk or bicycle ride through gardens, forests or beaches, or going skiing, are leisure activities that do not involve exposure to a lot of chemicals. Trees and plants help to clear some chemicals from the air and produce oxygen which also helps our detoxification systems work more effectively.

Stuff for Kids
With my children, I find one of the biggest issues in going out is dealing with them wanting treat foods. There are three ways I deal with this. Firstly, I take food with us whenever we go out so I don't need to buy anything. Secondly, if possible, I avoid going to places where treat foods are sold. For instance, I take the kids to a park rather than the mall, and choose a park that does not have a shop or ice-cream stand. We go to a library that does not have a cafe attached, to less popular beaches with no shops nearby, and I try and avoid taking the children to the supermarket. Thirdly, if we do have to go somewhere like the mall or the supermarket, then I may buy non-food treats such as a magazine or small toy.

How to Manage Social Situations
While food intolerances and allergies to substances such as nuts, gluten and dairy are becoming more well-known to the

general population, few people have even heard of things like salicylates and histamine. I have to confess, before I identified my intolerances, I did sometimes suspect that people who said they suffered from multiple chemical intolerance were just a bit over-sensitive about their health. I think sometimes the universe brings us experiences we need to have a better understanding of.

Most people will have no idea what you are talking about if you tell them you have a salicylate, phenol, histamine, glutamate or sulphur intolerance or even multiple chemical sensitivity. Unfortunately, these chemical intolerances are also quite complicated to explain and generally if you try people's eyes will just glaze over. As a result, I generally don't say anything unless I have to, or I just say we are allergic to something because it is easier for other people to understand. For example, when I am at the hairdresser, I state that I don't want any products in my hair because I am allergic to them. It is not a complete lie; I do react with allergy-type symptoms. It just makes life easier.

People, including your friends, relatives and partners will react in various ways when you tell them you have learned you have a chemical intolerance of some sort. My husband told me he thought it was a 'load of rubbish' when I initially tried to explain to him that I thought myself and my daughter had a salicylate intolerance. Some people will think you are being a hypochondriac, some might think you are just missled or misinformed, and others may flat out think you are crazy. My way of dealing with this is avoid the issue with them if I can or every so often point out evidence that may help them understand. I am aware that if you do not experience the symptoms of allergies or intolerances it can be very hard to understand how it works, and how uncomfortable and painful it can be. Before my intolerances became as severe as they are now, I used to find it hard to believe that someone could have an allergic reaction to peanuts just from smelling them. Now I break out in hives just from smelling coconut oil. We all want people to see things from our point of view, but sometimes we have to try and see things from the point of view of others first in order to help them understand.

Some people will accept and support you. Focus on these people and utilize their support because you will need it. Dealing with a food or chemical intolerance is challenging enough, but dealing with one that other people have no knowledge or acceptance of is even harder. You can also find support on-line through relevant forums and Facebook groups. Be gentle on yourself and others and aim to foster understanding all around.

If you do want to give a more in-depth explanation to someone here are some ideas you could try:

For salicylate intolerance: A simple explanation is that you (or your children) can't tolerate one of the chemicals found in most fruits and vegetables and in added food flavours and colours. A more involved explanation would be: "Some of my digestive enzymes don't work properly and I have trouble getting rid of a chemical called salicylate. Salicylates are found in all strongly coloured food, including natural and artificial colours, all strongly flavoured food, including artificial flavourings and all herbs and spices, and all fragrances both natural and artificial including essential oils." These explanations are not completely accurate nor do they cover all sources of salicylates, but they are enough to give someone an overview which is generally all people can understand.

For histamine intolerance: "I can only eat very fresh and quickly cooked food. Any food that has been stored longer than a day or two before being frozen, or that is slow cooked or fermented contains histamine." Again, this does not completely cover all sources of histamine but it gives a simple overview that others can understand.

For glutamate intolerance: "I can generally only eat fresh, natural foods with no processed ingredients."

If you have multiple chemical-intolerance like me, here's a combo explanation: "My digestive enzymes don't work properly and I can't detox certain chemicals. When they build up in my body I get allergy or irritable bowel type symptoms. I can only eat a small number of plain, fresh foods and react to all fragrances, both natural and artificial and most chemical cleaners and body products."

Managing Special Situations

Functions with alcohol if you are choosing not to drink: If you are with people you don't know very well then the easiest thing is simply to say: "I cannot tolerate alcohol. It makes me feel ill, but thank you for offering". If you have been a happy drinker previously, but choose to stop, then your friends and relatives may put pressure on you to join in the drinking. This can be hard. You could try something like: "I have found out that alcohol is one of the things that makes me feel sick so I am not drinking it at the moment, but thank you for offering." Another option is to get yourself a 'safe' non-alcoholic drink in a wine glass or something similar that you would normally have your alcoholic drink in. Then if someone asks you if you want a drink, you can gracefully say "no thank you, I already have a drink".

Going out for a meal: When you go out for a meal try to smile and laugh a lot because it helps to increase your tolerance levels. Let go of any worries about food, breathe deeply and enjoy yourself as much as possible as it is one of the best things you can do to reduce your reactions to higher chemical exposure.

My children and I react to so many different foods/chemicals that when we go out for a meal there is never anything completely 'safe' that we can eat. If you are doing an elimination diet you will need to either stay home or take suitable food with you if you can. When we go out for a meal, I call it a 'Free Meal". By this I mean we just eat want we want, enjoy it and deal with the consequences later. We try to avoid anything really high in the chemicals we react to or anything that will make us significantly ill, but apart from that we just savour it as a treat. This is alright for us because we don't eat out very often. Something else that can be helpful is to eat before you go out so that you do not need to eat much from the restaurant, or anything at all if it is a social gathering with finger food. If you have to eat out frequently for work, then you will have to become adept at asking for special meals to be made to keep your chemical levels low.

Soups and sauces often contain glutamate/histamine loaded stocks, and salicylate laden herbs and spices. It is usually best to avoid soups and either ask for no sauce, or for sauce to be served on the side, so you can choose not to have it, or to just have a taste.

Eat at clean, quality eating establishments only. If the visible area/serving staff are dirty, then the kitchen is probably worse.

Birthday and Other Parties: If it is a party for adults then I generally try and eat before I go and avoid eating snack foods/finger foods when I am at the party. If it is a party my children are attending then I either take suitable, safe treat foods for them, or approach it as a 'free day' and let them have what they want as long as it is not too high in chemicals they react to, or something that will make them significantly ill. As my daughter is older, I just let her manage herself at birthday parties, but for my son I attend with him and take some safe treats and then also let him have anything at the party that will not cause him too many issues. Usually, I remove the icing from birthday cake then let my children eat the cake. The cake is usually alright (not ideal, but not too bad) but the icing usually contains flavouring, colouring and numerous ingredients derived from corn which would cause significant problems. I also try to give the children plenty to eat before they go to the party (if they are not too excited to eat!) so that they are likely to get full sooner and eat less at the party.

Managing Partners/Spouses
In most cases one spouse or partner will identify or learn about food intolerances first. This is usually the mother or female because in most households women are still the primary caregiver of any children, and women are generally more interested in health issues (apologies for the generalisations). Generally, women seem to have more difficulties enlisting the support of their male partners than the other way round. This was the case for me so I asked for some advice from the Sue Dengate Failsafe Group on Facebook and below are some of the ideas people shared. They were directed at wives enlisting the support of their husbands, but most of these ideas would also work the other way round if that is the case with you. Most of the ideas follow the same theme of somehow helping your partner to visually experience the difference in behaviour or other evidence of reaction.

> ➢ When doing the elimination diet with your child/children, organise food challenges so that your partner can clearly see the before and after state of your child/children e.g., if your partner works full time plan

to have day 3 or 4 of the challenge fall on a day he/she is home with the children.

➤ Watch the Fed Up DVD (available from fedup.com.au) either together or by yourself but while your partner is around and can see and hear it.

➤ Ask your partner to take the children to the next dietitian's appointment

➤ If you have your children settled on a diet that largely eliminates chemicals they have issues with then go away for a week during normal routine time e.g. when they are attending school/kindergarten, and let your partner organise all their food while you are away i.e. do not leave any pre-prepared 'safe' food for your child/children. Having to manage the children around structured daily routines when their behaviour is going from bad to worse may help them to see the effect food has.

Just for interest: here is a quote for the sceptics who wonder how we can react to natural foods

"Although much attention has been paid in recent years to the adverse effects of food additives, naturally occurring food chemicals are a more insidious and more common cause of problems. Natural chemicals play a central role in the complex symbiotic relationship between animals and plants which has developed as a result of co-evolution. Plants are known to be capable of synthesizing an enormous range of substances important for their own survival and reproduction. Amongst these are a variety of anti-microbial and anti-parasitic agents, as well as chemicals which can modify the feeding behaviour of insects and higher animals. Not surprisingly, some of these substances can be toxic to humans if ingested in significant quantities."

The Role of Food Intolerance in Chronic Fatigue Syndrome. Robert H. Loblay, Anne R. Swain, in The Clinical and Scientific Basis of Myalgic Encephalomyelitis / Chronic
Fatigue Syndrome, B.M. Hyde, J. Goldstein, and P. Levine, Editors. 1992. The Nightingale Research Foundation: Ottawa. p. 521-538

Step 3: Eat the Right Things in the Right Way

I am not going to outline food elimination diets/protocols in this book. There are a number of good books with information about low chemical diets and it is a large subject. Read the Resources section in the Appendix of this book to see books I recommend related to low chemical diets. Also, as this book addresses multiple food/chemical intolerances I am not going to offer specific food lists because what you can or cannot eat will differ according to your specific sensitivities. What I am going to list here are some general diet guidelines that are applicable to everyone. These guidelines overarch what foods you eat and are to do with reducing inflammation and maximising digestion and nutrient intake. They are foundational guidelines for good health in general, but even more pertinent to us because our bodies are in greater need of healing.

Please note, these guidelines are ideals and may feel a little overwhelming, especially when you already have to avoid or eliminate so much from your life. My philosophy when it comes to diet (and life in general) is:

*Do your best
and don't sweat the rest*

We have enough to deal with without tying ourselves up in knots about eating the perfect diet all the time, and stress has as much of a negative impact on our health as consuming inappropriate food. This includes physical stress from not eating enough because you are trying to completely avoid all problem foods. When you are following an elimination diet you need to be strict and vigilant all the time, but once this identification phase is over, you can be a little more relaxed. Aim to follow the diet guidelines below as much as you can, but if you have the occasional piece of chocolate cake at a birthday party then just enjoy it and then get back on track as best you can.

I also advise making just one or two changes to your diet or lifestyle at a time. It takes longer, but it is much easier to manage and therefore you are more likely to be able to make the changes lasting ones that become new habits.

Avoid The Inflammatory Five: Sugar, Refined cooking oils, Gluten, Dairy and Alcohol

I hate to advise you to cut more foods out of your diet when you are probably already highly restricted in what you can eat. However, if you want to reduce your symptoms and allow your digestive and immune system to heal then it is best to avoid foods that are highly inflammatory and damaging, at least for a while. It is best to cut them out completely for a month or two if you can, but at least reduce your consumption of them to a minimum.

There are five types of foods that are the most inflammatory and damaging: Sugar, Refined cooking oils, Gluten, Dairy and Alcohol. Many of these foods are already off the menu for those of us with food and chemical intolerances anyway. Dairy is high in sulphur and fermented dairy foods like yogurt and cheese contain amines/histamine. Cheese can also inhibit the effectiveness of the Phenol Sulphur-tranferase (PST) enzyme which is essential to detoxing salicylates and amines. Alcohol contains histamine and most alcoholic drinks are also high in salicylates. Refined vegetable oils usually contain preservatives or hydrolysed lecithin which cause reactions in people with salicylate and histamine intolerance, and canola and rice bran oil contain sulphur. Wheat-germ is a histamine liberator.

Sugar
Diets high in sugar and simple carbohydrates such as white flour, white rice and potatoes often cause an overgrowth of yeast in your digestive system, and an imbalance of bacteria. This can lead to poor nutrient absorption and damage to your gut which can trigger or intensify food intolerances and chemical sensitivities. High blood sugar levels from a high carbohydrate diet can lead to the destruction of intestinal tight junction proteins thus causing or worsening leaky gut. Consuming sugar and simple carbohydrates increases inflammation in our body and brain which exacerbates any reaction symptoms, including brain related symptoms. It can also and increase pain.

Eating sugar lowers your chemical tolerance levels and increases your reactions: you react to more things with worse symptoms

This can be really hard to take on board, especially when one of the few safe foods for the chemically intolerant is white sugar and white rice. If you are going to eat white rice, then whole white rice is slightly better than rice flour. This is because it is absorbed at a slightly slower rate. It is also better to eat simple carbohydrates such as white rice with a protein containing meal as this helps to reduce high sugar insulin spikes. When potatoes and rice are cooked then cooled some of the potentially inflammatory digestible starches convert into beneficial anti-inflammatory resistant starch. This means that if you are going to eat potatoes and rice the best way to eat them is to cook them, cool them quickly in the fridge/freezer and then use them to make a salad containing protein. If you can eat them, consume wholegrains such as brown rice, oats and quinoa rather than refined white grains. We are born to like sweet tastes from our first sip of breast milk (or sweetened baby formula), and sugar is physically and emotionally addictive. Sugar cravings can also be a result of your chemical intolerance. When my chemical levels get high my blood sugar levels drop and become unstable, which makes me crave sweet, carbohydrate rich food. My daughter experiences the same thing. All this means that it can be very hard to reduce our intake of simple sugars, but here are some ideas that may help:

Tips to Overcome Sugar Cravings
Eat Less Sugar: The more sugar you eat the more sugar you will want. If you avoid eating sugar for about a month then its addictive grip on you will lesson. I have been eating a very low sugar/carbohydrate diet for several years now and my sugar cravings have dropped to just about zero. I still like sweet things. I don't like very sweet things like confectionery, icing and soda/fizzy drinks, but I still like cake, desserts and biscuits. I find I can go without these without too much trouble, but I also find that if I have some sweet foods, then I quickly start to want more.

Change Your Habits: Our tastes in terms of what we like and don't like are largely learned habits. Even though humans do have an inbuilt tendency to like sweet flavours, we also get into habits of eating sweet things. Breakfast is a good example of this. Most of us get used to, i.e., into the habit of, eating sweet foods for breakfast such as cereal and fruit. We feel disinclined to eat savoury foods for breakfast because it is not what we normally have. I now have the opposite issue. I have been eating a savoury meal for breakfast for a number of years so the thought of eating something sweet for breakfast now feels unusual and unattractive to me. My habits have changed, and yours can too.

Get Plenty of Rest: When we get tired, we tend to crave sweet food. Aim to get enough good quality sleep every night, rest when you need to, and avoid pushing yourself too hard mentally or physically.

Relax: Like when we are tired, when we get stressed, we crave sweet food. See the section on Stress earlier in this chapter for practical ideas on how to stay relaxed.

Find Safe Sources of Comfort: We often eat sweet foods as a form of comfort when we are feeling sad, stressed or even angry. Identify non-food ways of gaining comfort when you feel overly emotional. Some ideas for ways to feel better without food include:

Give or receive a hug or cuddle (from a human or a furry friend)

Talk to a friend

Get some exercise - it produces feel-good endorphins. Go for a walk with a friend so you can chat and move at the same time

Have sex

Get a massage

Watch a funny movie (without the chocolate and popcorn)

Create something

Eat a nutritious diet: Low nutrient levels can cause our bodies to crave fuel which we usually interpret as sugar. Eating a low-carbohydrate diet consisting mainly of fresh meats and fish and fresh vegetables is the best way to keep your body well-nourished and provide the raw materials for producing the feel-good neurotransmitter serotonin.

Follow The Sun: Exposing your eyes to natural light early in the day helps set your circadian rhythm correctly and stimulates the release of hormones that help you feel positive and alert. Vitamin D, which your body produces when your skin is exposed to sunlight also boosts mood.

Get socially savvy: One of the hardest things about trying to reduce your sugar intake is managing friends and family helpfully tempting you with sweet offerings and gifts. Let people know that you have an illness and sugar makes it worse so you are trying to avoid eating sweet foods. Talk about things you like other than sweet foods ie avoid saying "I wish I could have a chocolate bar" because this makes other people think that you really do want a chocolate bar and will offer you one or buy you chocolate as a gift because they think it is what you like. Set your focus and consequently the focus of those around you, on non-food things that you enjoy. Talk about things you like that are not connected to food e.g. "I'd really like to see that movie . . ." Or "I really enjoy reading the . . . magazine", or "I would really like to try [fishing, sewing, Salsa dancing, tennis . . .]. This keeps your focus away from food and gives other people information about alternative things you like and ideas for non-food related gifts.

Interesting Tip: Saffron, one of the few spices that is low in salicylates, is high in manganese which helps regulate blood sugar and metabolize carbohydrates (it also helps you absorb calcium). Make sure you buy authentic Crocus sativus from Crocus flowers though as sometimes cheaper alternatives are sold as saffron. Buy saffron from somewhere with a high turnover to ensure that it is fresh – a specialty ethnic food shop may be a better source than a supermarket.

Kids and Carbs
While I try to keep the amount of refined sugar and sweet foods that my children eat to a minimum, they do still eat white rice as a major part of their diet. Ideally, I think it would be good for them to eat an animal protein and vegetable based diet, but it is nearly impossible to get a child to eat like that. If your children can tolerate wholegrains then try to give them those instead of refined grains. However, many children with digestive and detoxification issues have difficulty processing wholegrains because of the fibre or higher sulphur or chemical content. If they can only eat refined grains like white rice try to include it in savoury meals to fill them up, and keep sweet baking to a minimum.

Definitely make very sweet sugary foods a once or twice a week treat only. This in itself can be hard in our sugar saturated society where lolly jars sit on bank counters and supermarket checkouts are lined with confectionery. I try to avoid going to places where sweets are available as much as possible. I go to the supermarket without my children and keep cake and sugary foods to special occasions like birthdays. It can be very hard to say no to children, but I have found that if you consistently stay strong when you say no that in time your children learn that no means no, and you don't change your mind, and the tantrums and pleading etc become less. I have also found that it helps to set clear boundaries at the beginning. For example, before going into a shop that has treat food available, I will say "Today we are not buying treat food. We are only buying . . ."

It also helps to talk to your partner about treat foods and try and form agreed guidelines around what the children can have and when. This can be a hard conversation to have especially if you are not both on the same page concerning your children's chemical and food intolerances. If you have a partner who does not completely accept your children's intolerances, then choose a time to discuss it when you are both calm and free from distraction. Let your partner know you would like to come to an agreement that you are both happy with, ask your partner what they think, and try to come to the best compromise you can.

Refined/Hydrogenated Vegetable Oils
Most cooking oils are highly refined including rice bran oil, corn, soy, peanut, canola, safflower, and also sunflower unless it is truly cold pressed. To make vegetable oils, nuts and seeds are pressed or chemical solvent extracted (the most common form of extraction), degummed, bleached and deodorised to produce a product that is colourless, odourless and tasteless. This strips the oil of most of its nutrients. Citric acid (which usually contains corn and glutamates) is often used as a degumming agent. As vegetable oils are polyunsaturated they are very sensitive to light and heat. In most cases even cold pressed vegetable oils are actually heated, and then most are packaged in clear plastic bottles. The exposure to heat and light causes the oils to go rancid and creates damaging trans fats and free radicals. Oil is a good solvent so it is highly likely to leach chemicals out of the plastic bottles it is stored in (always store fats in glass containers). As a result of all this most vegetable oils are highly inflammatory, toxic and can cause damage to your blood brain barrier. The only exceptions to this are oils that are expeller pressed at low temperatures, protected from light, air and heat during production and sold in dark glass bottles. Even carefully produced vegetable oils are high in omega 6 fatty acids though which are also inflammatory in large amounts. For those who tolerate salicylates, good quality, unrefined, cold pressed olive oil sold in dark glass bottles is usually okay because it contains mainly monounsaturated fats. Store it sealed in a dark cupboard and use it only for low temperature cooking.

Margarines and spreads made from refined oils go through even more processing producing even more damaged fats. Avoid anything which contains hydrogenated or partially hydrogenated fats as they are high in disease promoting trans fats. Processing aside, soy and canola oils are usually made from genetically engineered crops and often contain pesticide residue. Soy and corn oils contain glutamate.

The best fats/oils for cooking, depending on your intolerances, are monounsaturated or saturated fats such as: butter, ghee, lard, tallow, coconut oil, cacao butter, unrefined olive oil and sustainable palm oil.

Gluten
I am aware that there is a lot of debate about whether wheat and gluten are harmful to everyone. This debate is also fuelled by the fact that they are nutritious foods, and also because they are products which are the mainstays of most western economies. They are also versatile, readily available and taste nice. However, I think there is enough research available to promote caution about consuming them on a regular basis. Some resources you may want to read on this topic include: *Good Health in the 21st Century* by Dr Carole Hungerford, any of the books by Dr Rodney Ford and *The Paleo Approach* by Sarah Ballantyne PhD.

Even if you do not have a diagnosed allergy or sensitivity to gluten, it is wise to avoid consuming it because it is highly likely to cause damage to your gut. Here are a few reasons why:
- ➢ The specific lectins found in wheat (wheatgerm agglutinin WGA), as well as alpha-amylase/trypsin inhibitors found in gluten containing grains, have been shown to cause the release of inflammatory chemicals from intestinal immune cells

- A high concentration of wheat lectins can lower the pancreas's ability to produce digestive enzymes by up to 70%
- Wheat is high in fructans which are a type of starch not easily broken down by humans and may feed the bacteria involved in small bacterial overgrowth (SIBO)
- Consumption of wheat can reduce nutrient uptake and production and lead to nutrient deficiencies
- Wheat gluten is a source of free glutamate

Dairy
Consumption of cow's milk and cow's milk products can cause the following issues:

Mucus: Most milk contains a protein called BCM 7 which is known to increase mucus production in your respiratory and digestive systems. Excess mucus in your gut can decrease nutrient absorption. It is definitely wise to avoid milk if you have a cold.

Insulin Spikes: High levels of insulin promote inflammation. When you drink milk your pancreas releases a lot of insulin.

Toxic pollutants: Dairy products have been shown to contain some of the highest levels of environmental pollutants such as flame retardants and dioxins. These toxins can damage our immune system. Part of the reason toxin levels are so high in milk is because they accumulate on plants which the cows eat and then the cow stores the toxins in its fat tissues. The animal then uses stored fat to produce milk and the accumulated toxins are freed into the milk.

Disrupted digestion: cow's milk contains protease enzyme inhibitors which can create or worsen a leaky gut. The protease inhibitors can prevent you from digesting proteins effectively. These undigested proteins can activate your immune system causing inflammatory damage to your gut.

Low iron levels: consuming cow's milk can decrease your absorption of iron and irritate the intestinal lining causing chronic blood loss

As a general rule if you are going to consume dairy then fresh, plain, ideally organic, whole milk, cream or unsalted butter is best (iodized salt contains sulphites). A2 milk generally causes less issues than A1 milk. You can buy A2 milk at most supermarkets now, and sheep's and goats' milk are also A2. However, if you have any kind of significant gut issues, I would recommend avoiding dairy altogether, at least for a while.

If you are worried about getting enough calcium if you do not eat dairy products, then there are other ways to ensure your body has all the calcium it needs. If you are eating mainly fresh meat and eggs and as many vegetables as you can then your calcium intake should be adequate. Meat and fish supply your body with small amounts of calcium as well as the protein and vitamin A it needs for calcium utilization. Cooking stews or casseroles with meat on the bone helps to up your calcium intake. Bones are also high in sulphur, but I find I can tolerate one meal a day of meat cooked on the bone if my chemical levels are low. Fish roe is another source of calcium. Most vegetables contain some level of calcium absorbed from the soil. Lettuce, parsley and other leafy greens, especially the darker leaves, are a source of calcium. They are also a good source of vitamin K1 and magnesium which are two important co-factors for calcium utilisation. Try adding leafy greens to an omelette, or soup, or green smoothie for breakfast. If you can tolerate them, chickpeas are high in calcium and many other nuts, beans and seeds also contain this mineral. The calcium is most absorbable if they are soaked and/or sprouted before being cooked.

You can make a calcium supplement from dried, ground eggshells. Eggshells contain calcium carbonate and you can buy eggshell calcium in supplement form, however it is easy to make your own, and then it also has no problematic additives. At least one study has demonstrated that the calcium carbonate from eggshell powder is absorbed as well as or better than purified calcium carbonate

To make eggshell calcium powder, first wash the eggshells thoroughly, but try to keep the inner membrane in place as this contains nutrients like collagen, glucosamine, and hyaluronic acid. I just scrub the outside of mine with a brush and wash out the insides, but if you want to be extra thorough you can wash them and then put the shell in a pot of boiling water for 10 minutes. I wash and dry the eggshells as a I use them. You can store unwashed shells in the refrigerator and then wash larger batches at once. If I did this, I would boil them as well. Dry and sterilize the eggshells by putting them in a dish in an oven heated to 100 degrees Celsius for 10-15 minutes. Lastly, grind the dried eggshell to a fine powder in a clean coffee grinder and store the powder in an airtight glass jar in a dark cupboard.

One teaspoon of eggshell powder contains about 800-1,000mg of calcium. Eggshell powder can cause minor digestive upset so it is best to start taking small amounts and build up to about 1 teaspoon a day for adults, ¼-½ a teaspoon for children. Some people recommend taking it with food, and some people recommend taking it on an empty stomach. I cover both bases and take ¼ teaspoon with lunch, ½ a teaspoon on an empty stomach in the afternoon and ¼ teaspoon with dinner. You can mix it with food or water. I add it to baking for my children. Take calcium and iron supplements several hours apart from each other. Taking a vitamin D3 supplement with the eggshell powder will aid absorption of the calcium, as will taking it with magnesium or high magnesium foods.

One of the reasons many people need extra calcium is because there are many factors in our modern lifestyles that cause our bodies to lose or poorly absorb calcium. A diet high in sugar and starchy carbohydrates causes your body to leach calcium from your bones in order to balance its pH levels. Excessive consumption of meat can have the same effect. Sugar also inhibits your body from metabolising calcium effectively. Phosphoric acid in fizzy drink/soda, and fructose and fruit acids in fruit and fruit juice can inhibit calcium absorption in your digestive system. Phytates in grains, soy and beans, and phosphorus from a diet very high in animal protein, including milk, can also decrease calcium absorption. Stress causes your body to lose calcium as does excessive sodium intake because your kidneys excrete calcium with sodium. Significant fluoride intake from fluoridated water, or foods made with fluoridated water, can lead to fluoride replacing calcium in your bones causing them to become brittle and weak.

Vitamin D and magnesium are just as important for bone health as calcium, as is weight bearing exercise. Going for regular, relaxing walks in the sun and eating a low carbohydrate/low sugar diet with as many vegetables and legumes as you can should help you maintain adequate calcium levels, and keep your bones and teeth strong.

Alcohol
Even small amounts of alcohol can burn the tips of the villi in your small intestines. The villi are important for secreting digestive enzymes and absorbing important nutrients. If the alcohol contains gluten even more damage can be caused. When alcohol is drunk in excess or on an empty stomach it can accelerate the development of a leaky gut. Alcohol is also

high in sugar which will feed bad bacteria in your gut increasing the risk of an imbalanced microflora environment in your intestines. All this decreases the amount of nutrients you absorb and create via your digestive system, and in addition to this your body has to use significant amounts of vitamins and minerals to process the alcohol you drink. This can lead to nutrient deficiencies.

Alcohol is broken down into Acetaldehyde in your body which is toxic and has been shown to damage DNA. Ingesting alcohol significantly increases the amount of work your detoxification systems have to perform and can lead to liver damage. It also dehydrates your body which increases histamine levels and puts pressure on your body's detoxification systems.

General Food and Diet Guidelines

Eat Adequate Protein
Protein is essential for the supply of amino acids. Those of us with food and chemical intolerances are likely to have gut damage that inhibits our uptake of amino acids meaning that we may need to eat more to get the same amount of nutrition as people with healthy digestive systems. Either that or consider taking an appropriate digestive enzyme to help you to digest protein more effectively. Animal proteins are one of the best sources of b vitamins including thiamin (vitamin B1), riboflavin (vitamin B2), pantothenic acid, folate, niacin (vitamin B3), vitamin B6 and B12. Red meat contains the highest amounts with lamb containing the most, although chicken breast is good source of vitamin B6. B Vitamins are essential to the effective functioning of our body's detoxification and anti-oxidant processes. Animal protein and fat also contain a highly absorbable form of vitamin A especially liver, eggs, butter and fish (if you have trouble with chicken eggs, try duck or quail eggs instead). Fish and

chicken are high in selenium and also contain vitamin E. Chicken thigh is high in zinc. However, while animal proteins are very nutritious, too much protein can cause an imbalance and lead to the loss of minerals from our bones and teeth. Eating animal proteins with vegetables helps to prevent this though. Meat also contains moderate to high levels of glutamate. Rabbit and turkey are highest in glutamate, and grain-fed animals and fish may also produce meat/flesh higher in glutamate. Lamb contains lower levels, as do eggs. When I consume glutamate, I experience early morning insomnia. At one stage I was eating chicken 2-3 times a day and was experiencing chronic early morning insomnia. When I reduced this to no more than one serve of chicken a day, I no longer experienced insomnia on a daily basis. This may be because chickens are typically fed a grain and soy-based diet.

This prompts the question: How much protein should I eat?
My ambiguous answer is much as you need to and an amount that feels right for you. The standard guideline is that protein should make up about ¼ of each meal. When you are severely limited in the number of foods you can eat though, you just have to do the best you can, and everyone has individual protein needs that fluctuate from time to time depending on our metabolism and levels of activity. When my chemical sensitivities first flared to extreme levels I could eat hardly any vegetables and no fruit. I also could not eat legumes or whole-grains because the sulphur content made me break out in painfully irritated rashes on my face and neck. However, I also couldn't eat a lot of refined grains because the high carbohydrate level made me break out in cystic acne. Consequently, I ate a lot of animal protein – to be exact I ate a lot of chicken thigh fillets because that was the only meat I didn't react to, apart from the insomnia issue which I worked out later. This wasn't ideal, but it was the best I could do at the time. High animal protein levels may lead to your body leaching minerals from your bones and teeth, but so does the

consumption of sugar and high carbohydrate foods and in my mind, it is better to eat nutritious meat than nutrient devoid sugar. Eating vegetables with animal protein helps to balance out your body's pH levels, and prevent the leaching of minerals from your bones and teeth. As soon as my tolerance levels increased, I added more vegetables to my diet and decreased the amount of animal protein.

The Fish Question
Fresh, clean fish is a good source of protein and anti-inflammatory omega 3. Many people avoid eating fish either because of fear of histamine issues or toxic contamination. Small fish at the bottom of the food chain are likely to contain lower levels of contaminants, but still only eat fish if they are sourced from an area with relatively low pollution levels. Salmon is often fed dyes along with antibiotics so check how it is farmed and what it is fed carefully before consuming it. As long as the fish you eat is gutted, filleted and stored in ice as soon as it is caught and then you eat it the same day then the histamine levels should be low. Washing the fish before you cook it also helps reduce contaminants and histamine. Frozen fish that is processed in western countries is usually low in histamine, but it may have been dusted with corn starch to keep it from drying out. Avoid shellfish because it is not gutted and is usually high in histamine and other preservative chemicals such as sulphites.

What About Vegetarian Diets?
The main source of vegetarian protein is grains, nuts, seeds and legumes. Most wholegrains, nuts, seeds and legumes are high in sulphur, and many also cause issues for those with histamine intolerance. Most nuts and seeds are high in salicylates, and grains, nuts, seeds and legumes are all high in anti-nutrients that can make them hard to digest, especially for people with damaged digestive systems. Animal proteins contain higher levels of readily metabolised nutrients than

vegetarian sources of protein and few problematic chemicals. If you choose to eat a vegetarian diet due to ethical reasons then you will have to do the best you can, but you will need to be even more conscious of what you eat in order to consume sufficient nutrients to keep your body in good health. In particular, you will have to monitor your levels of Vitamin B12, iron and zinc which are essential for immune function and can be difficult to obtain in optimum amounts from a vegetarian diet, and even more so from a vegan diet. My research leads me to believe that an omnivorous diet is the healthiest one for humans. This doesn't mean eating a lot of meat necessarily, it is healthiest for vegetables to form at least half of your diet, but eating naturally raised animal proteins at least five times a week gives your body good amounts of the nutrients it needs for health and healing.

Prioritise Nutrition
As we have such a limited diet, those of us with food and chemical intolerances need to be far more careful about choosing to eat the most nutritious food we can. Base your diet on fresh vegetables, meat, fish and eggs. If you tolerate them you can add in 1-2 serves of wholegrains or legumes a day, but many of us can only tolerate refined grains which are too high in sugars and should be restricted as much as possible. Fibre is important to cleanse your digestive system and feed beneficial bacteria in the gut, but vegetables are the best source.

Minimal water-based cooking is best, for example stews, soups, casseroles, steaming and poaching. Food that has been browned from grilling, frying or baking is high in amines/histamine and often contains carcinogenic compounds. Cooking eggs for extended periods on high heat causes the cholesterol in them to oxidise, and destroys some of the nutrients. Over-cooking protein denatures it, destroys some of the heat sensitive amino acids and can make the protein more resistant to digestive enzymes. Cooking vegetable oils at high heats can cause them to oxidise. Stir-frying is alright but keep the food moving and use the traditional stir-fry method of cooking the ingredients in a little water and then just adding oil at the end for flavour. Cook foods until they are just cooked through or just softened in the case of vegetables. Eat fruit and vegetables raw on a regular basis if your digestive system can cope with it (raw foods can be harder to digest than cooked). Blending raw foods into a smoothie can make them easier to digest.

Once your tolerance levels increase, prioritise including more nutritious foods i.e., instead of thinking "Yay! now I can eat chocolate occasionally" think, "Yay! now I can include some more vegetables in my diet and make my meals more interesting." Some good foods to include once you can tolerate higher levels of chemicals include green bananas, legumes, sunflower seeds and darker leafy greens. If you have problems with histamine, you could try eating cooked green bananas (unripe yellow bananas) which are lower in amines, though being unripe they will be higher in salicylates. Green bananas are lower in sugars than yellow and so may be better tolerated by those of us who have trouble metabolising carbohydrates, but they are high in resistant starch so only eat them cooked and even cooked they may cause issues for people who have difficulty digesting fibre. Green bananas are a good source of vitamin B6, vitamin C and potassium. The resistant starch they contain also feeds probiotic bacteria in your gut, reduces inflammation in your colon, helps increase your body's insulin sensitivity, and helps your body absorb more minerals such as calcium.

Legumes, especially lentils, are a good source of folate. Salicylates may have a blocking effect on the uptake and utilisation of folate meaning that an extra high intake may be beneficial to those of us with chemical detoxification issues.

Extra folate may particularly help with chemical sensitivity symptoms associated with the brain and nervous system such as brain fog. Most legumes (avoid red beans) contain anti-inflammatory and anti-histamine properties. Soaking legumes in very warm water with a small amount of baking soda overnight before cooking helps to remove most of the nutrient blocking compounds such as oxalic acid.

Sunflower seeds are high in vitamin E which can be another nutrient that is hard for those with food intolerances to get from foods. Sunflower seeds are best brought raw, as fresh as possible and stored in the freezer. They are easier to digest if ground so either grind them before storing them in the freezer or add the whole seeds to a smoothie.

Leafy greens such as the Cos lettuce, fresh parsley, fresh coriander and the dark outer leaves of Iceberg lettuce are a good source of magnesium, folate and chlorophyll, and help feed beneficial gut bacteria. Chlorophyll is the green colouring in foods. It is an anti-oxidant and binds with toxic metals and some carcinogens to inhibit their absorption in your body. Lettuce can be lightly cooked like spinach, chopped and added to rice or noodle dishes, or used as a cup or wrap and filled with mince, chicken or hummus.

Some high nutrient foods can be added to meals in small amounts as flavourings such as saffron, fresh squeezed lemon juice, fresh parsley, fresh coriander, fresh chives and fresh garlic. I would like to make a note about saffron though. Saffron is a good source of vitamin C, folate, calcium and beta-carotene (vitamin A). It is generally listed as having low/no salicylate content. When I tried a small amount, it did seem to help relieve my intolerance symptoms. However, when I tried eating it with one or two meals a day, after a few days I started to experience the following symptoms: constant gnawing hunger, low blood sugar, brain fog, increased skin itching and disturbed sleep. These symptoms generally indicate a salicylate issue for me and I would expect that due to its strong colour saffron would contain salicylates. Whether it contains salicylates or not, it appears that for us chemical intolerance sufferers a little of this spice on occasion may be helpful, but it might be best to avoid eating it regularly.

It is also a good idea to prioritise anti-inflammatory foods and anti-histamine foods such as those below:

Anti-inflammatory foods
- Chamomile Tea (it is also relaxing and may help promote sounder sleep - use loose leaf tea as teabags may contain chemicals such as sulphites)
- Chickpeas
- Chickweed (herb commonly found growing wild in home gardens)
- Fresh Coriander
- Fresh Garlic
- Fresh Parsley
- Fresh Turmeric
- Leafy greens
- Lotus root (Indian)
- Olive oil
- Omega 3 Fatty acids – fish, walnuts, grass-fed beef and lamb
- Zucchini/Courgette or marrow (if you have a salicylate intolerance use large zucchinis or marrow and peel it thickly)

Anti-histamine foods
- Apple (contains histamine lowering quercetin)
- Celery (contains histamine lowering quercetin)
- Chamomile Tea (it is also relaxing and may help promote sounder sleep - use loose leaf tea as teabags may contain chemicals such as sulphites)

- ➢ Chickweed (herb commonly found growing wild in home gardens)
- ➢ Chives (contain histamine lowering quercetin)
- ➢ Fresh Coriander (contains histamine lowering quercetin)
- ➢ Foods high in vitamin C (vitamin C is a natural anti-histamine)
- ➢ Fresh Parsley (prevents histamine release and is high in vitamin C)
- ➢ Fresh Turmeric (prevents histamine release)
- ➢ Green Beans (contain histamine lowering quercetin)
- ➢ Green Pea and Chickpea Sprouts (these are rich sources of natural DAO enzyme which helps you process histamine. See below for how to grow and eat them at home)
- ➢ Legumes (contain histamine lowering quercetin)
- ➢ Lemon juice (high in vitamin C and quercetin)
- ➢ Lettuce (contains histamine lowering quercetin)
- ➢ Lotus root (Indian)
- ➢ Olive oil (contains quercetin)
- ➢ Omega 3 Fatty acids – fish, walnuts, grass-fed beef and lamb
- ➢ Saffron
- ➢ Whole Buckwheat Groats (the whole groats are very high in histamine lowering quercetin, the flour contains some quercetin but much less)
- ➢ Zucchini/Courgette or marrow (if you have a salicylate intolerance use large zucchinis or marrow and peel it thickly)

How to Grow and Eat Pea and Chickpea Sprouts – A Natural Source of Diamine Oxidase Enzymes (DAO)

Diamine Oxidase helps your body to process histamine. People with Histamine Intolerance often have a lack of, or poor functioning, DAO. Green pea and chickpea sprouts contain natural DAO (they are also a good source of vitamin A and C, folic acid and oxygen). I cannot tolerate fresh or frozen green peas (or any legumes) due to their sulphur, glutamate and lectin content, but I thought I would try the pea sprouts smoothie outlined below. I found that when I drank the pea sprout smoothie it appeared to reduce my intolerance symptoms especially the itching in my skin. I did still appear to have a small reaction to the glutatmate in pea sprouts, but research indicates that the level of glutamate and aspartate in legumes drops when they have been sprouted. When I introduced the pea sprouts to my diet, I thought I might try adding some chickpea sprouts to the mix for extra calcium, and then sunflower sprouts for vitamin E. However, when I tried having just one or two of each of these sprouts together, I had an immediate severe reaction. My mouth started burning and my throat started to swell. Fortunately, I was able to control the reaction by taking baking soda. Raw legumes and seeds are high in citric acid. I believe that it was this that I reacted to. Legumes also contain significant amounts of phytoestrogens and A-Linolenic Acid. A- Linolenic Acid stimulates moderate histamine release, and excess oestrogen can be inflammatory and immunosuppressive.

In light of all this, I do not personally consume pea sprouts. I have included the recipe below for the pea-sprout smoothie outlined by Dr Janice Doneja. You can assess what the risk-benefit balance of them would be for you personally.

Method for making DAO rich pea-sprout smoothies
- Use dried green peas (the best source of natural DAO) or chickpeas designed for sprouting
- Rinse the peas or chickpeas in clean water
- Cover the rinsed peas with more clean water in a bowl or sprouting jar, add about ¼ teaspoon of sodium bicarbonate and soak them for 12-24 hours. Peas, like all legumes, contain lectins. Lectins can damage your intestinal lining, but soaking the peas/chickpeas

overnight in water with sodium bicarbonate added, and then sprouting them for the 9 or 10 days as per recommended below should deactivate most of the lectins.

- Drain off the soak water and put the peas in a sprouting bag or jar with a mesh sprouting lid (the lid just makes rinsing easier – if you don't have one you can simply put the peas in a glass bowl or jar to sprout and use a sieve to rinse them)
- Place the peas in a dark place such as a drawer or cupboard, or wrap the jar in a towel. The dark environment increases levels of DAO in the sprouts. Keep them at room temperature.

- Sprout the peas for 9-10 days (no more). Rinse them with clean water 2-3 times a day to keep them clean and moist, but shake off any excess water or store the mesh lidded jar upside down to let excess water drain out.

- Only eat mature sprouts that have sets of two leaves
- Blend the sprouts whole in a blender to make a smoothie. The sprouts need to be eaten raw and pulverised to release the DAO. Eat the whole sprout.

- Consume the smoothie just before a meal to help process histamine in that meal or consume small amounts over the day to help lower histamine levels generally.

Start with small amounts, but you can build up to about 1 cup a day. Leftover sprouts can be stored in the refrigerator in a sealed container with a paper towel or microfiber cloth on the bottom to absorb excess moisture. Sprouted legumes contain some histamine and accumulate higher levels of histamine the longer they are stored. For this reason, I advise making staggered small batches rather than one large batch i.e., start a new small batch of sprouts every 2-3 days. Sprouting smaller batches every 2-3 days also prevents the sprouts becoming crowded in the jar. When the sprouts get crowded, they start to rot.

Eat Organic Where Possible
Generally, it is better to choose organic foods and products. I say generally because sometimes the salicylate content of organic foods is higher, for example I can tolerate commercial celery, but experience symptoms of salicylate sensitivity when I eat organic celery. However, salicylates are usually higher in genetically modified foods as well. Some chemical pesticides contain lead and arsenic, and cadmium is a contaminant in phosphorus-based fertilizers. Organic grown foods are often higher in nutrient content and usually lower in heavy metal contaminants, but organic farmers still use natural pest control products that may cause issues for those of us who are particularly chemically sensitive. Whatever food you choose to eat wash it thoroughly before consuming it. I also prefer to eat lightly cooked fresh food. Cooked food is easier to digest for many people and there is a higher risk of bacterial and parasitic infection from raw and stored/reheated food.

Organic meat and eggs are generally preferable, or at least meat and eggs from free range, grass fed animals. Free range animals that are allowed to forage naturally are exposed to less chemicals from medications and are less likely to be fed genetically modified feed. Meat and eggs from free range animals contain higher levels of omega 3, vitamin K and anti-inflammatory conjugated linoleic acid (CLA). In saying that, I can eat commercial chicken but I had a strong reaction to a brand of free-range chicken I tried presumably because of something it was fed.

Grains
It is best to buy grains whole so that you can rinse them thoroughly in hot water before cooking them to remove chemicals, heavy metals, bacteria and parasites. It is also best to cook grains and pasta in a lot of water and then discard the cooking water to further cleanse them of contaminants. Due to the physiology and growing conditions of rice it can accumulate up to ten times more arsenic than other grain crops, but rinsing and cooking it in plenty of water can remove over 50% of this contaminant. Brown rice flour, rice bran, rice-based sweeteners and rice bran oil are not cleansed in this way and so are likely to contain arsenic. The processing of white rice will remove many contaminants. If you are going to use flour buy organic flour (wheat and all gluten-free flours) as it is less likely to contain chemical and heavy metal pollutants and usually does not have sulphites added to it.

Chew Your Food Thoroughly
When you chew your food, you break it down and enzymes in your saliva begin to digest your food, especially carbohydrates like fruit, vegetables and grains. Breaking food down thoroughly makes it easier to digest, and can reduce the level of reaction to it. Chewing your food thoroughly also releases more energy from your food and more nutrients. This means you get maximum value from the food you do, and can, eat which is necessary for those of us on very restricted diets. We need to get all we can out of the food we are able to eat.

Eat Adequate Amounts
It is important to eat enough food regularly to keep your blood sugar levels stable and to feed your brain a constant supply of energy. However, the act of eating releases inflammation in your body and overeating puts a strain on your digestive and detoxification systems. The best way to

fuel your body for health and healing is to eat three nutritious meals a day with your biggest meal at lunch and a lighter meal in the evening. Leaving several hours between eating allows for your insulin levels to fall and helps your body to produce and utilise insulin appropriately.

When you graze on small meals through the day, especially if those foods are high in carbohydrates such as sugar, fruit, grains and starchy vegetables like potatoes, your insulin levels remain elevated. High insulin levels promote inflammation in your body and over time decrease your body's ability to absorb and utilise insulin which is called insulin resistance. When you develop insulin resistance, insulin levels in your body remain high and cause further inflammation. Aim to make each of your meals high in nutrients and satisfying with plenty of unprocessed natural fats and protein so that it sustains you until the next meal. If you do need to eat a snack between meals, then try to have a protein-based snack rather than a sugar based one, for example nuts, homemade chicken soup, hummus or coconut chips. The need to snack is mostly the result of habit, modern societal norm, or meals not being nutritious enough.

Avoid eating within 3 hours of going to bed. Eating less in the evening allows your digestive system to rest and heal while you sleep. Having significant amounts of food in your intestines when you go to bed can also cause disrupted sleep. The act of eating raises histamine. If you experience histamine intolerance then it may be best to try and eat just three meals a day. If you have a slower metabolism, you can even try eating just two meals a day - a large, high nutrient brunch and then an evening meal. However, I do know of at least one person who has histamine intolerance and reflux and they find it best to eat several smaller meals over the day. You may need to experiment to find out what works best for you.

What About Children?
Children tend to be more active and require food more often. However, for children as well it is best to aim for three high nutrient main meals with protein-based snacks at mid-morning and mid-afternoon. I say aim because between children's tendency for fussy eating and frequent exposure to other food providers (play-dates, birthday parties, grandparents etc) it is much harder to keep them to a stable, balanced diet so remember, do your best and don't sweat the rest.

Keep Your Salt Intake Low
Salt, sodium chloride, seems to cause problems for me. I am not exactly sure why. At first, I thought it was the type of salt I was using. Himalayan pink salt is high in sulphur which I react to, as is the grey unrefined sea salt or wet salt. I don't like the idea of using normal refined salt as I have read that we do not absorb or utilise it well because its crystalline structure is deformed during high heat processing, and iodized salt contains sulphites. I currently buy a cleaned natural sea salt, but even that causes me problems. I have read that sea salt contains glutamate. In The Paleo Approach Sarah Ballantyne notes that recent research has shown that higher levels of sodium chloride in the diet causes increased inflammation. In Ayurvedic philosophy salt is heating and may cause skin issues such as rashes and acne in susceptible people, but rock salt is considered less heating than sea salt. Salt can also be very irritating for your gut - when you put salt on your skin it can cause dryness, itching and even burning and it can have the same effect on the lining of your intestines. Higher levels of salt from chips or crackers give my son digestive upset and reflux.

Do we need to consume salt?
There are varying opinions on this. We can gain sodium and chloride from vegetables including celery and lettuce.

Prehistoric man and many traditional societies did not, and do not, add salt to food with no obvious detrimental effects. However, while there is some scientific evidence that high salt intake can cause or aggravate health issues there is also evidence that low salt intake may also cause issues such as disturbances in cholesterol and calcium metabolism.

My advice would be to find a balance. If you are not able to eat take-away meals and processed foods then your salt intake is probably already significantly lowered as these foods are very high in salt. If you are making most of your own food from scratch and adding salt to taste then your salt intake is probably at a happy balance, but avoid high salt foods like crackers, chips, bread and canned foods. Try and use a natural, unrefined salt, preferably rock salt. I add salt to some of my meals, but not all, and I find I don't tolerate anything highly salted like rice crackers. It took me a while to get used to the taste of food without salt, but now I prefer some without salt, though I still like to lightly salt any meal with fish, rice or noodles.

Interesting note: if you have a strong desire for salt and salty foods your zinc levels may be low.

Eat The Right Fats
It can be a little challenging finding fats to use when you are chemical intolerant especially if you are dairy intolerant as well. My children and I can only really use fresh fats from meats as canola and rice bran oil are too high in sulphur, most vegetable oils contain antioxidants which can be a problem and we also react to palm shortening. If you can find a quality dripping or duck fat source they can be alright, but try and buy them as fresh as possible and use them as quickly as you can as they can contain amines. A couple of things I have found helpful are:

- use silicone bakeware as you do not need to grease it

- cook meat in a little water.
- When you cook meat in a little water it helps to draw out the fat in the meat to lubricate it while cooking. For example, when I make a stir-fry or noodle dish, I cook the meat in a little water in the wok first letting the water cook off as the meat cooks. Leave a little of the fatty water behind, remove the meat, then cook the vegetables/noodles in the fatty water and lastly add the meat back in.

- leave as much fat on your meat as possible, but not chicken skin if you are sensitive to amines.

My research leads me to believe that it is perfectly safe to eat natural saturated fats from meat and eggs. Fat is an essential nutritional element. It is a good source of energy and nutrients. It also helps to keep your skin lubricated from the inside which is helpful for those of us who cannot use many skin creams externally. Research shows that natural saturated fats are healthier than processed unsaturated fats like those from vegetable oils as the latter cause high levels of inflammation in our bodies and are lower in nutrients. Fat from fish is also very beneficial for our bodies, but avoid stored fish and fish skin if you have an issue with amines. I can get away with eating a small amount of very fresh fish every few days and I try to do this to keep up my levels of omega 3. Fried foods are very unhealthy. The high heat often oxidises and damages the fat used, which is usually a refined vegetable oil that is inflammatory anyway. Fried foods also contain chemicals shown to damage your colon tissue and the DNA of your colon cells.

Something to be aware of is that fats are histamine releasers which means that when we eat them our bodies release histamine from our mast cells. Some types of fat cause high increases in histamine, and some types release very little.

Here is a summary:
Very high – Arachidonic Acid: Offal is high in arachidonic acid. Chicken eggs are also relatively high, but for comparison duck eggs are relatively low.

High – Linoleic Acid: found in significant quantities in flax seeds, sunflower seeds, nuts, chicken fat, duck fat, egg yolk and seed-based oils.

Moderate – A Linolenic Acid: found in flaxseeds, chia seeds, hemp seeds, soybeans, walnuts, herbs, micro herbs, seed and legume sprouts, broccoli, cauliflower, zucchini, avocado, onions and butter. A Linoleic acid is beneficial in preventing inflammation, but paradoxically also leads to moderate histamine release.

Moderate-low – EPA and DHA essential fatty acids: found in fish and grass-fed protein.

Low – Medium-chain Triglycerides: found in coconut oil, coconut milk and breast milk. Oleic Acid: found in olive oil, avocadoes, lard and nuts like macadamias. Stearic Acid: found in meat, coconut and milk.

What to Eat
It is healthiest to form the base of your diet around fresh vegetables and fresh animal proteins. This is true even for most people who are free from food and chemical intolerances. Focus on using fresh, unrefined fats to cook with. If you have no fructose intolerance you can add in a few fresh fruits. If you have no sulphur issues you can add legumes and gluten-free whole grains.

Although eating this way can be challenging when it is very different from those around you, in time your tastes and habits change and it does get easier (although when my stress levels start to climb, I find it harder to 'go without' the treats that others can eat). Take strength from the knowledge that eating this way will not only help decrease your chemical intolerance symptoms, but also improve your overall health. In addition, it can improve your appearance since high sugar and alcohol consumption causes your skin to sag and wrinkle, and is the most common cause of excess weight. Focus on what you gain and how much better you feel when you eat a healthy, anti-inflammatory diet.

Reintroducing Foods
When you begin to re-introduce foods that you haven't eaten for an extended period of time proceed very gently. A guideline may be that the first time you re-try a food have a teaspoon or less, and then wait at least 7 days before trying another teaspoon. Once you've done this for a few weeks you can try having two teaspoons, once every 7 days for a couple of weeks. After this you can try rotating a very small serve of the food every 4 days (96 hours). I know this can seem like a hard and tedious process, but taking it slowly is the best way to get your body to accept the food once more. You can try one different re-introduced food every 2-3 days for example try some green beans on Monday, some chamomile tea on Wednesday and some fresh coriander on Saturday and then repeat this the following week. I would not recommend re-introducing more than three different foods a week though. Re-introducing foods in this way is even more effective if you combine the re-introduction of the food with meditation, visualisation and brain retraining techniques (see Stress Trauma above for more information on this)

Celebrate each step forward no matter how small. You may only be able to tolerate five green peas once a week, but that is a start, and it is an extra five green peas worth of nutrition and variety that you were not getting before.

Rotating Foods

Once you can eat enough different foods it is a good idea to eat a rotational based diet. This takes a bit of thinking ahead and planning, but it can help keep your tolerance levels up and reduce your risk of developing another food sensitivity. When we eat the same foods repeatedly day after day we can develop an intolerance to them. You could aim to rotate foods on a four day basis, for example if you have carrots with dinner then do not eat carrots again until at least dinner-time four days later. You do not have to be too strict about it though as you don't want this to become a source of stress. Just aim for as much rotating variety in your diet as possible.

Desensitisation

I have not seen desensitisation discussed much in chemical intolerance circles. I came across a summary of it randomly one day and then came into contact with someone who had tried it successfully. From the report I have, this desensitisation is mainly used for salicylate intolerance, but there are noted instances of it being used successfully for amine/histamine intolerance also. I do not know the science behind it and I do not know how or why it works, but it works for me. The report I read cites numerous testimonials from people who had tried this desensitisation protocol for their children or themselves and experienced very positive results.

I had the information for a long time before I tried it myself for various reasons. The principle behind it is quite simple, but almost the reverse of what we with chemical intolerances normally think. Basically, you consume increasing amounts of salicylates on a frequent regular basis over 3-5 days and if you start to react you consume more, rather than less. The theory is to keep giving doses before your body has a chance to react. It feels a little strange, especially if you have been avoiding salicylates for a long time and I think that you need to prepare yourself mentally as well as organisationally, and try it at a time when you can stay focused and relaxed. The desensitisation protocol is simple. You start by taking an initial dose (portion of salicylate containing food) that is small enough that it wouldn't on its own cause a reaction. You then take a second dose which is double the first before your body has a chance to react. Thus, if you would normally react within one hour then take a dose every 30 minutes, or if you would normally react within 3 hours then take a dose every 90 minutes. However, generally, most people find it works to give a dose every 2 hours. I found it helpful to use a timer to remind me to take the next dose.

How often and for how long you need to continue this process depends on your individual sensitivities, but most people find that the following plan works.

Basic Desensitisation Plan
Day 1: Take the initial dose early in the morning and then double the previous dose every 2 hours. Do this throughout the day until bed-time.

Day 2: Start with an initial dose early in the day that is the same as what you finished with the previous day. Continue to take doses every 2 hours and continue to increase each dose by half or double. You can start to level out the dose if you reach a point that you want to be desensitised to. For example, if you want to be able to tolerate 4 pieces of moderate salicylate fruits/vegetables a day then you can stop when your consumption has reached that level.

Day 3: If your consumption of salicylates has reached the level that you want then continue to consume salicylates at that level over the course of this and every subsequent day.

Especially for the first few days, continue to spread out your consumption of salicylates fairly evenly over the day.

Day 4 and following. You will need to maintain your salicylate consumption each day at about the level you have desensitised to. Most people find that if you go significantly below that level or above that level then you will once again experience withdrawal or intolerance symptoms.

For the first day of desensitising at least it is easiest to use only one food so that you can be fairly accurate about dose levels. Once your tolerance starts to build you can be a little more flexible and introduce a greater variety of foods. I would recommend having a few small doses of the food you are going to use over the two or three weeks before starting the desensitisation process if it is not a food you have consumed for some time as per the note on food reintroduction above. This gives the body a little time to 'get used to it' before beginning to consume significant amounts.

Some suggested initial foods and their salicylate content per 100gms are:

- Mango (0.11mg)
- Apples (approximately 0.4mg) NB apples may be problematic for some people due to other phenols
- Cucumber (0.78mg)
- Peaches (fresh 0.58mg, tinned 0.68mg)
- Apricots (2.58mg)

Some people also use honey. You could try diluting 2 teaspoons of plain honey (not Manuka or fragrant) in 2 tablespoons of warm water and then take ¼ teaspoon of this solution as the initial dose. As the dose increases over time you could change to taking straight honey. One mother who performed this desensitisation protocol with her child cut up a honey sandwich into 16 squares and gave one square as the initial dose.

Some foods not recommended for desensitisation as they may cause issues due to other components:
- Carrot
- Apples (numerous phenols)
- Strawberries (benzoates, tannins)
- Oranges (amines)
- Pineapple (amines)
- Grapes (glutamates, tannins, possible sulphites)
- Rock melon (amines)
- Passionfruit (amines)
- Tomato (amines)
- Raspberries
- Watermelon (tannins)
- Kiwifruit (tannins)
- Bruised apples, peaches or apricots (tannins)

When I undertook my desensitisation, I wanted to avoid sweet foods like fruit and honey because too much sugar causes me to get cystic acne. I had been wanting to try taking flaxseed oil to get some more healthy fats in my diet because I was currently eating very little fat, so I decided to use that for the desensitisation along with moderate to high salicylate vegetables like cucumber, zucchini and butternut squash. However, I towards the very end of the desensitisation process I learned that flaxseed contains substantial amounts of fats that release high levels of histamine in your body. Although I tried desensitising to histamine after I desensitised to salicylates, I still seemed to have issues with histamine causing skin itching and eczema for me. As I result, I stopped taking flaxseed. I also stopped eating chicken on a regular basis for the same reason. Chicken fat, along with soybeans, and chickens are often fed soy-based feed, also contain substantial amounts of fats that release high levels of histamine. Duck fat does as well. It appears I had finally found the reason these foods caused problems for me when by most accounts they should have been fine. I did a bit of a combination of food reintroduction and desensitisation. By that I mean that I introduced a small amount of the foods first before starting the desensitisation process. Thus, I had small amounts of flaxseed, chickweed and cucumber occasionally over a few weeks prior starting desensitisation and then introduced single serves of new foods like zucchini and butternut squash and rotated them in with the flaxseed and cucumber. I am aware that most people don't eat chickweed. It has about the same low-moderate level of salicylates as fresh coriander which would be a more accessible alternative. Herbs like chickweed and fresh coriander have anti-histamine properties as well as being very nutritious.

I am a very sensitive, super-responder. I worked on the principle of taking the next dose when I started to notice reaction symptoms from the previous dose so initially, I took doses every 20-30 minutes. As my symptoms began to settle, I started to extend the time between doses.

My Desensitisation Plan
Day 1: I started taking one drop of flaxseed oil and then doubling the dose approximately every half hour. As I had to take doses so frequently, by lunchtime I had already taken a high daily dose of flaxseed oil and so I switched to eating a chunk of peeled cucumber every 30-45 minutes and then adding some fresh chickweed to that. For dinner I had some peeled zucchini and then went back to taking the cucumber and chickweed until bed.

I was having mild reaction symptoms by the afternoon including mild vision blur and itchy skin on my neck and inner elbows where I get eczema.

Day 2: I continued to take a 'dose' every 30 minutes until midmorning and then I took a dose every 45-60 minutes (I was not strict). I took a combination of foods. Mainly about a 2.5 segment of peeled cucumber and 2 sprigs of chickweed, but I mixed that with butternut pumpkin with breakfast, 3 teaspoon doses of flaxseed oil and a serve of peeled zucchini for dinner. I treated myself to salmon and avocado sushi for lunch.

I experienced quite strong skin flushing and itching around the middle of the day, but I did sit in the sun for an hour or so in the morning which usually causes those symptoms as well as salicylates. For the rest of the day my skin experienced mild itching and prickling on and off but less than Day 1.

Day 3: I slept more soundly than usual and woke with my skin feeling relatively settled. My mood was very positive. This was possibly because my symptoms were low and I was starting to feel hopeful that this might work, but anxiety is one of my salicylate toxicity symptoms. I followed a similar protocol in terms of food dosages to day 2 except that I took the doses every hour (approximately). I also added in spraying rose water onto my skin several times a day.

Rosewater is probably low-moderate salicylate. I wanted to try it because it was said to soothe irritated skin and eczema, and because it was a relatively safe first fragrance to reintroduce. I had 4 blueberries for supper and spent the evening with someone wearing strong fragrance. I experienced mild skin irritation symptoms from the fragrance, but not as strong as I normally would.

Day 4: Followed a similar protocol in terms of food and hourly doses as per Day 3. I upped the level of my salicylate intake a little by having basmati rice for dinner. My intolerance symptoms had only been occasional mild itching on the back of my thighs and neck. I was in the sun quite a bit that day also though, and my stress levels had been slightly raised.

I also felt a little nervous. I seemed to be improving, but I felt anxious that at some point I would 'crash' and the symptoms would all return with a vengeance. I had tried so many things in the past which seemed to help in the beginning, but then after a while caused problems or stopped working. I worked on releasing this fear and anxiety and taking one day at a time, because the stress would raise the level of my intolerance symptoms and issues.

Day 5: Same as Day 4.

Day 6: As per Day 4 and 5 but I also introduced coconut oil. I wanted to introduce coconut oil for two reasons. One as a histamine desensitisation, and secondly because I wanted to introduce more fat into my diet as I was eating almost none apart from some from the teaspoon of sunflower seeds I had with breakfast and from the chicken I usually had for lunch.

Coconut seemed the most beneficial choice for me. It was recommended as one of the few beneficial fats for my Ayurveda Pitta dosha, and has been shown to improve digestive, liver and immune function. I introduced it using the same desensitisation protocol as for salicylates and started with a small taste and then increased the amount every 30 minutes. Further reading had indicated that consumption of flax oil causes high levels of histamine to be released from mast cells due to the linoleic acid content, so my aim was to reduce the amount of flax seed oil I was taking and replace it with the coconut oil. While coconut oil contains amines, it causes virtually no histamine release from mast cells.

At my first dose of coconut oil, I experienced significant

intolerance symptoms within about 10-15 minutes so I took the next dose quite soon after. By late morning my skin was itching and my eyesight was blurring. During the afternoon the symptoms eased to mild itching and my eyesight cleared. However, by evening my skin was very sensitive and I had several very small whiteheads around my mouth which is a common salicylate intolerance symptom for me. From late afternoon on I stretched the doses to 45-60 minutes apart. My teeth and gums were also aching mildly.

Day 7: As per day 6 but took about ¼ teaspoon of coconut oil every 30 minutes until about mid-morning and then every 45 minutes until lunchtime and then every 60 minutes for the rest of the day. I slept well the night before, although I did have an Epsom Salt and sodium bicarbonate footbath before bed. When I started taking the coconut oil in the morning my symptoms become quite strong. My skin was itching and very sensitive. I was also experiencing frequent urination, aching teeth and a mild sore throat. By mid-afternoon my symptoms were mild.

Day 8: Took about ¼ teaspoon coconut oil approximately every 60 minutes from waking. Food routine is now three meals plus morning and afternoon tea as per the Maintenance Diet schedule below. Symptoms have been mild all day today, about the same level as an average day on an avoidance diet.

Day 9: Slept soundly. When I awoke my skin felt settled. This was the first time in months that I had awoken free from itching skin. Food as per Maintenance Diet. Took approximately ¼ teaspoon coconut oil every hour until early morning and then every 90 minutes. Very low symptoms all day until late afternoon when my stress levels and level of fatigue grew high.

Day 10: As per Day 9 but taking just over ¼ teaspoon coconut oil every 90 minutes from waking. Very low symptoms all day until evening when I experienced some mild prickling and itching of my skin. I was very fatigued though from a very busy day.

Day 11: As per Day 9 but taking just over ¼ teaspoon coconut oil every 2 hours from waking.

Day 12: Maintenance Diet with peeled fruits and vegetables. Swapped morning teaspoon of flaxseed oil for one teaspoon ground golden flaxseed.

Over the following week I started having zucchini with the peel on and replaced the flaxseed oil with ground golden flaxseed.

After about a week on the maintenance diet my day-to-day symptoms issues were lower than they had been on an avoidance diet, and some cleared completely. I was sleeping soundly through the night most nights, my eyesight was clear. I was feeling energised, positive and generally very healthy and happy. However, I was still having mild issues with itchy/prickly skin and eczema which are caused by histamine intolerance for me. As I mentioned previously, the histamine desensitisation did not appear to have worked as well as the salicylate desensitisation and so I stopped consuming some of the foods that caused high levels of histamine release such as the flaxseed, and chicken meat and fat. My skin was generally settled and clear of eczema and itching once I did this. Over time I also increased the amount of coconut oil I was consuming from ½ teaspoon doses to 1 teaspoon doses without adverse effects.

My Maintenance Diet
(please note: this is for reference only and not intended as a

prescription for everyone. This is what suits me, but I have included it to give others a guide to work from. This is my base diet, but I do vary it from time to time. I use it as a reference to maintain my salicylate intake at about the same level. I eat largely according to the suggested diet for an Ayurveda Pitta dosha because I find that this helps to keep my skin settled).

On rising
½ teaspoon of coconut oil. 2 drops of iodine rubbed into wrists. One probiotic capsule with water. Every 2-3 days: zinc sulphate rubbed into wrists. 30 minutes after probiotic and before breakfast: low dose iron supplement

Breakfast
Split mung dahl and oat porridge with one serve butternut pumpkin, 1-2 teaspoons soaked sunflower seeds and 1/2 teaspoon coconut oil. Vitamin D supplement and selenium supplement every 2-3 days.

Morning Tea
Smoothie with about 2.5cm chunk cucumber (initially skin removed), 4 sprigs fresh chickweed or coriander, ½ teaspoon coconut oil. Optional: 1 cup of chamomile tea

Lunch
White Basmati rice/rice noodles with legumes or lamb or duck egg or chicken thigh or fresh fish. One serve zucchini (peeled initially)/asparagus and selection of celery, green beans, lettuce, and/or cabbage. ½ teaspoon coconut oil. ¼ teaspoon eggshell powder.

Afternoon Tea
Smoothie with 1 sweet apple (peeled initially) or 2.5cm chunk cucumber, 4 sprigs fresh chickweed or coriander, ½ teaspoon coconut oil, ½ teaspoon eggshell powder.

Dinner
Split mung dahl and white Basmati rice/legumes with rice noodles. One serve zucchini/butternut squash/asparagus and selection of celery, green beans, lettuce, and/or cabbage. ½ teaspoon coconut oil and ¼ teaspoon eggshell powder.

Bedtime
2 drops of iodine rubbed into skin, magnesium sulphate footbath or solution rubbed into skin

For me, desensitization worked/works. As far as I am aware it is not a cure, but rather another management protocol. Instead of managing your intolerance by avoiding salicylates, you manage it by taking regular doses. You need to continue taking the same level of salicylates each day. If your intake becomes significantly higher or lower, then intolerance symptoms return. However, managing my intolerance by taking regular doses of salicylates gives me much more freedom in terms of what I eat, what I use for self-care, and being comfortable in public spaces.

I have been following this protocol for some time now and my salicylate intolerance symptoms remain lower than they were on an avoidance diet. My eczema is now minimal most of the time and I experience much less skin itching issues. The 'crash' I once feared has not happened and I do not think that it will. The desensitisation seems to remain constant. At one point I spent time sitting by an indoor swimming pool watching my children swim. After an hour my head was aching, my sinuses were burning and I was beginning to feel nauseous. I felt like I had been sitting in a gas chamber and my chemical toxicity levels were very high. I experienced significant chemical intolerance symptoms, but I continued to follow my high salicylate Maintenance Diet. The only thing I did for detoxification support was drink a teaspoon of baking soda in water twice a day for the first day of exposure, and then half a teaspoon in water twice a day the next day. Within 2-3 days the symptoms/issues had cleared and I was once again relatively symptom free on the Maintenance Diet. I was thus able to work through an instance of increased exposure, but maintain the high salicylate tolerance I had attained through desensitisation.

Step 4: Avoid Chemicals (Without Avoiding Life)

As I mentioned in Step One, focus on removing environmental sources of chemicals first and foremost. For some people this may be enough to significantly reduce or eliminate their symptoms and they may not have to eliminate many or any foods. Most sources of environmental chemicals can be eliminated without too much change to your life; it is just a matter of identifying alternative products to use. Although in saying that, identifying products that are safe to use, especially when you have more than one chemical sensitivity, can be very challenging. Hopefully this book will help make it easier for you.

When I first became aware of my chemical sensitivities, I struggled to find suitable options that would allow me to do the things I once normally did. I couldn't even find skincare that was suitable let alone make-up. Even the natural cleaners such as white vinegar that I had been using were now a problem, and finding a suitable toothpaste was a costly and time-consuming endeavour. After a lot of searching and trialling I have found options that work but it took me many, many stress-full months. Thus, to save others that time and expense I have made a list here of all the things that should be alright to use if you have any combination of sulphur, salicylate, amine or glutamate sensitivity, or if you suffer from multiple chemical sensitivity. Before I begin the list though, there are a couple of things I would like to note.

To Get Better Avoid All Synthetic Chemicals

Obviously, your first priority will be to avoid the specific chemicals you react to, however, because chemical sensitivities are all connected to low functioning detoxification and immune systems it is helpful to reduce your exposure to all chemicals which would stress your body. In order to give our bodies space to heal and 'unload' we need to reduce our exposure to synthetic fragrances, chemical estrogens (xenoestrogens), petrochemicals and chemical-based cleaning products as much as possible. Be aware that anything which causes your hormone levels to fluctuate may increase your chemical sensitivities which includes exposure to synthetic hormones as well as natural events such as puberty, pregnancy, menopause and stress. If you do not have a salicylate sensitivity then you can probably use many truly natural skincare and cleaning products, but if you are sensitive to salicylates you will need to avoid anything containing plant or herbal extracts and oils including essential oils.

Personal Care

It took me quite a long period of trial and a lot of error to identify what I could safely use to wash and groom myself. Hopefully this list will make this process much faster and easier for you.

Dental Hygiene

Toothpaste

There are some low salicylate toothpastes available, but they do cost much more than regular toothpaste. I have tried both the Alfree and Cleure brands and found them both pleasant to use, and they do not appear to cause any issues for my children or I. However, we use a very small amount and rinse our mouths out after brushing. Alternatively, you can use plain baking soda (sodium bicarbonate). I used this for many months. It takes a while to adjust to the taste, but I liked how clean and fresh it made my mouth feel. I also found that it whitened my teeth subtly and that my teeth felt very smooth and clean. The other plus of using baking soda to brush your teeth is that it is mildly anti-bacterial and alkalising making it an effective mouthwash as well. Sodium bicarbonate also helps your body to detox chemicals.

I have read concerns about baking soda being too abrasive. Before I identified my food intolerances and significantly reduced my exposure to the chemicals I am intolerant to my teeth were very sensitive and when I tried using baking soda to clean them it made my teeth and gums ache. However, once I had been avoiding my chemical triggers for a while and had begun taking the supplements I refer to in this book then my teeth were no longer sensitive and I could use the baking soda. I used it regularly to brush my teeth twice a day for a year or so and did not experience any problems.

To use baking soda as toothpaste I kept a jar of sodium bicarbonate in the bathroom, wet my toothbrush slightly, dipped it in the jar to coat the brush then brushed my teeth as normal. Instead of rinsing it out straight away I took a couple of sips of water then swished the solution around in my mouth and gargled it a few times as a mouthwash before spitting it out. I recommend using high quality, additive and aluminium free sodium bicarbonate for personal hygiene uses rather than the sort you get at the supermarket. See the appendix for recommended brands, or purchase it from a natural health foods store.

Interesting Tip: Gargling activates the vagus nerve at the back of your throat which stimulates your gastrointestinal tract and improves the functioning of the gut-brain axis. However, to be truly effective you need to gargle long enough and deep enough for it to be a bit challenging. Try gargling three times each morning and evening after you have brushed your teeth.

Dental Floss
Flossing your teeth helps to remove the plaque that can build up between your teeth as well as any food debris stuck there. However, most dental floss contains mint flavouring or synthetic flavourings which are a problem for most of us with chemical intolerance. Even if you can find an unflavoured floss most dental floss is made from nylon, a synthetic fibre derived from petrochemical products, or polytetrafluoroethylene (PTFE). PTFE is commonly known by the brand name Teflon. It belongs to a class of perfluorochemicals (PFCs) which are thought to be carcinogenic, are suspected hormone and endocrine disruptors, are associated with neurological problems and suppress the immune response. There are natural dental floss products available which are usually made from silk, but most contain essential oil flavourings.

You could try using colour-free, unbleached natural cotton thread to floss your teeth (be aware that most commercial sewing thread is made from nylon). This may be hard to obtain, and it may leave fibres between your teeth so brush carefully afterwards. There is a product available called a water flosser which uses plain water to clean between your teeth. This is a costlier option. The traditional Ayurveda practice of oil pulling is said to help remove debris from between teeth as well as toxins from your body. It takes about fifteen to twenty minutes each morning, but it can be a relaxing, meditative practice. I have done it in the past, but have not had the time opportunity since my son was born.

Type of Toothbrush
Plastic contains many chemicals that may cause problems especially to those of us with sensitivities and using it to scrub your teeth makes it likely that some of the plastic will wear off and enter your mouth. If you use a plastic toothbrush, then choose one with white/non-coloured bristles and rinse your mouth out very thoroughly after brushing your teeth. If you are going to gargle after brushing your teeth, then I would recommend rinsing your mouth carefully first and then gargling with a fresh solution of baking soda and water. Alternatively, you could try using a natural material toothbrush such as one with a bamboo handle and biodegradable polymer bristles. I use bamboo toothbrushes from Go Bamboo. They look very plain compared to the high-tech plastic brushes that you can buy now but I find that they work and last very well.

Breath Freshener
As mints are off the menu for most of us, when I want a quick breath freshener I add a pinch of baking soda to some water, swish it round my mouth for a minute or two then either swallow it (as I'm rushing out the door normally) or spit it out.

See the Recommended Products and Recommended Resources sections in the Appendix for more information on dental floss, water flossers and bamboo toothbrushes.

Skincare
I tried a number of different options for cleansing my face from natural cleansers to basic soaps to baking soda and oil cleansing. My skin was so sensitive and reactive that everything I tried caused problems until I started using a microfiber face cloth with just water. It took my skin a little to get used to it, but after a couple of weeks it was fine. I use an Enjo face glove.

All natural moisturising lotions contain plants oils and/or plant extracts which contain salicylates. Most non-natural moisturising lotions contain petrochemical derived mineral oil, which I react to, and other chemical ingredients which may not necessarily cause reactions but which have been shown to cause other health issues. The only moisturising agent I found that I didn't react to, and felt comfortable using, was refined jojoba oil. Even though I don't noticeably react to it I use it very sparingly, but it does keep my face hydrated and smooth. Jojoba oil starts to solidify like wax in cold temperatures so in winter I keep small amounts in a wide mouth jar, scoop out a little of the 'wax' with my fingers and melt it in my hands before applying it. I rarely use moisturiser on my body. I found that when I stopped using soap on my skin and only cleaned it with the microfiber cloths and water then it became less dry and was okay without moisturiser. You can increase your skin's hydration internally by drinking plenty of clean water, eating unrefined natural fats and taking a quality omega 3 supplement (see Step 4 below).

Rose water is low-moderate in salicylates so may be tolerated by some. I started using rosewater when I began my desensitisation protocol and I never noticed any issues with it. It is beneficial for skin. It also acts as fragrance, and can be used as a deodorant. Rosehip oil is likely moderate-high in salicylates, but may be tolerated by some. You could mix a small amount of rosehip oil and jojoba oil together.

Andrea Rose produces a range of salicylate and fragrance-free skincare products as does Cleure. The Fed-Up website also lists options which others have found suitable. See the Recommended Products list in the Appendix for more information.

Hair Care

There are some hair care products available that are suitable for those of us with chemical sensitivities. Andrea Rose produces a range of salicylate and fragrance-free hair care products as does Cleure. The Fed-Up website also lists options which others have found suitable. I personally use Eco-store fragrance-free shampoo and conditioner. This is derived from natural ingredients, but seems to be processed enough to be safe. See the Recommended Products list in the Appendix for more information.

Here are some other hair care and styling tips for the chemically intolerant:

Get a Dry Haircut

While it is very nice to get a head massage with your salon shampoo treatment, for those of us with chemical intolerances salon hair products can be a huge trigger. Barber's and while-you-wait type hairdressers will cut your hair without washing it first. I wash my hair at home before I go. Also, remember to request that they do not put any product in your hair. It is fine to get it blow-dried without styling products. You could take your own shampoo/conditioner/styling product to the hairdressers. Note that salons which use a lot of products in the hair-cutting process will also have high concentrations of chemicals in the air even if they are not being put directly on your scalp and hair. While-you-wait salons in shopping malls often have an open end with no door which is helpful for reducing the amount of salon product chemicals in the air.

Opt for Simple Style

It is best to have your hair cut in a style that does not require a lot of hair-styling products to get it to look good. It is also best to avoid chemical treatments such as permanent waves and hair dyes. Embrace the real you and look for styles that suit your hair's natural features.

Wash Less
Unless you use a lot of product in your hair, which is now unlikely since I think almost all manufactured hair products contain natural or synthetic chemicals that cause reactions, or your hair gets coated with dust or dirt regularly, then it only needs washing once or twice a week. If you normally wash your hair every one to two days, then it will take a month or so for it to settle into being washed less often, but after that you will find that it gets less oily and more manageable as well as softer and less dry. When I had my hair short I washed my hair with water only in the shower every day, but only shampooed it once or twice a month as it needed it. When I first started doing this my hair started to look like it needed a wash by about day three, but after several months it stayed fine almost indefinitely. If you want to read more about this then search on 'no poo hair method' on the internet.

Hair Styling
As far as I have been able to see almost all manufactured hair care products except certain shampoos and conditioners contain natural and/or synthetic chemicals that cause reactions. I have found four 'safe' hair styling products that you can make at home.

Refined Jojoba oil: You can rub a small amount of jojoba oil in your hands and then smooth it onto your hair to calm fly-aways and frizz. Use a very small amount though or your hair will become oily and weighed down. Apply it like you would a serum.

Dry shampoo: Basically, the idea of dry shampoo is to use an oil absorbing powder to absorb the oil on your hair and scalp. You can use dry shampoo to touch up your hair between washes. As 'dirty' hair often holds its style better than just washed hair you can also use dry shampoo to make your 'dirty' hair presentable and easy to style. You can use just about any form of absorbent starch that you can tolerate - cornstarch (contains glutamates), tapioca or arrowroot starch (use organic and ensure it is free of sulphites) or cocoa powder if you have dark hair and no sulphur or histamine issues. Simply brush the starch powder onto the oily parts of your hair, rub it in, shake, brush or comb out any excess powder, and then style your hair.

Salt Spray: You can use the following sea salt spray to add volume to your hair, style shorter hair or create beachy waves. I find this works well, but the salt in it irritates my sensitive skin.

Mix together one cup of hot water, 2 tablespoons of Epsom Salts, ½ teaspoon of sea salt and ½ teaspoon of chemical free conditioner until all the ingredients are dissolved. Pour the mix into a spray bottle for storage and easy application (glass if you can find one).

Spray this on damp hair and scrunch with a towel for loose beach waves or spray it on dry hair or hair roots for added volume. You can also wash your hair the night before, spray it with the sea salt spray then French braid it or twist it into a bun on top of your head (avoid using a hair tie or you'll get a hair tie kink). Leave overnight and the next morning when it is dry spritz your hair lightly with a little more salt spray and take out the bun/braid. You can lightly spray your hair again and scrunch it once it is down to add extra volume and hold.

Texturising Setting Spray: This spray gives your hair texture and also sets it a little like hairspray. Like the Salt Spray, you can use this to add volume to your hair, style shorter hair or create beachy waves. I prefer this styling spray to the Salt Spray as it does not irritate my skin.

Mix together 1/2 cup of hot water, 1 teaspoon of Epsom Salts,

1 tablespoon of white sugar, 1 teaspoon of vodka or colloidal silver (as a preservative – note that vodka contains histamine) and ¼-1/2 a teaspoon of chemical free conditioner (optional) until all the ingredients are dissolved. Pour the mix into a spray bottle for storage and easy application (glass if you can find one). You can leave out the conditioner if you have oily hair.

Spray onto dry hair and scrunch the hair until the spray dries, or spray onto dry hair and then use a curling iron to create curls/waves. You can also use it as per the Salt Spray above to create easy morning hair by braiding or twisting your hair up overnight.

Deodorant
Finding a deodorant/antiperspirant that is free from reaction causing chemicals can be challenging. It should at least be free of colour and fragrance including essential oils, and it is also advisable to use a deodorant that does not contain aluminium. There is a list of suitable options on the Fed-Up website and both Cleure and Andrea Rose stock chemical and fragrance-free deodorants (see Recommended Products – Personal Care). There is also a chemical free range called Crystal Stick which makes a fragrance-free option. You can buy this at most natural health stores or online. If you use a store bought deodorant product re-check the ingredients each time you buy it as manufacturers may change ingredients from time to time.

You can make your own deodorant using baking soda. You can either use plain baking soda or blend it with a little corn or tapioca starch. The baking soda helps kill odour causing bacteria and the starch absorbs perspiration. For a while I used plain baking soda. I kept some baking soda in a wide mouthed jar in the bathroom with a small round Enjo make-up remover microfibre pad in the jar which I used to dust on the baking soda. I found that this worked reasonably well to stop odour, but that it sometimes left white marks on my clothes especially if I perspired a lot.

I now dissolve a Chrystal Stick deodorant block in colloidal silver to make a liquid, then pour some into a spray bottle and use that. I find that it is reasonably effective as a deodorant and I prefer it to the baking soda as it is quicker and easier to use, and easy to carry with me and reapply as needed. Sometimes I add a weak solution of cooled chamomile tea to give it a slight fragrance. If you are going to do this add the tea to small batches of the deodorant and use it as quickly as possible to prevent bacteria breeding in the tea solution.

I have also seen Milk of Magnesia, which is magnesium hydroxide solution, recommended as a deodorant, but I have not personally tried this.

If you can tolerate it then rose water could be used as a fragrant deodorant. It is low-moderate in salicylates. I have tried this, but did not find it very effective. It would be better combined with something like the Chrystal Stick deodorant or added to the spray mix I described above.

Keeping your chemical levels low may reduce your need for deodorant anyway. Before I identified my chemical intolerances and reduced my exposure to the chemicals, I was reacting to I used to suffer from very strong body odour and excessive perspiration. Now I don't seem to have these problems. I also have not experienced this issue since increasing my salicylate intake through desensitising.

Hair Removal/Shaving
For Women
As I have a salicylate sensitivity and had problems with finding a soap I didn't react to and razors free of moisturising

strips I tried using an epilator. I found the epilator alright to use. However, epilation, along with waxing and plucking, can cause physical trauma to your skin. Physical trauma stimulates inflammation and the release of histamine. After a while I noticed that my symptoms increased on the days I used the epilator. Although advertising claims that epilation will give you weeks of hair free skin, I find that I have to do it at least once a week, plus it is much less painful to epilate when your hair is very short. To reduce the 'trauma' I would epilate one leg one day and the other one the next. I do like the fact that epilation results in soft regrowth which is nice on your legs, and also means you can use it on your thighs, bikini and arms with no irritating stubbly regrowth. Theoretically you can use an epilator on your underarms, but I found this too awkward and painful and I still shaved under my arms. Waxing may be okay as it generally lasts several weeks meaning that the exposure to physical trauma induced histamine release is less frequent. The wax used may be low in salicylates and other chemicals (you will need to ask as they vary from salon to salon), but the soothing cream applied afterwards is likely to be high in them so either take your own cream to put on, or ask for just an ice-pack to soothe the area that has been waxed.

If you wish to shave then you will need to either use an electric shaver, or find a soap/shaving cream free of reaction causing chemicals and also razors that either have no moisturising strip or one that is free from problem chemicals. If you are going to shave in the shower turn the temperature down as heat can stimulate the release of histamine. Using a microfiber exfoliating glove after shaving, epilating or waxing can help smooth flaky skin and reduce the amount of moisturiser needed. Use minimal amounts of a chemical-free moisturiser or refined jojoba oil to soothe any dry skin.

For facial hair removal, the chemical-free options include

waxing, plucking, using a plucking coil such as a Bellabe, or IPL/laser hair removal. All these options cause physical trauma to your skin and the release of histamine. I tried using a Bellabe, but found it quite tricky to use and it left my sensitive skin irritated and inflamed. I have fair facial hair, but I have quite a lot of it and several thicker darker hairs around my upper lip and chin. I have always been self-conscious about it so I decided to try IPL laser hair removal. As my hair is fair it had to be waxed first so the treatment felt like having my face waxed and then tattooed. My skin was inflamed for about a week afterwards, but only about as much as it normally is after I have it waxed. The hope was that after about 4-5 treatments most of the darker, longer hair on my face would be permanently reduced/removed and I will only have to have a maintenance treatment once a year from then on. However, after about 4 treatments I had noticed no change in the amount of hair on my face and was finding the treatments too painful so I decided to stop.

2021 Addendum: One of the new trends in facial hair removal is microblading. Microblade shavers do not have any added moisturising strips so are a good option for people with chemical intolerances. I have personally been microblading my face, arms and upper legs for a couple of months now and am very happy with the results. It is quick and easy and exfoliates the skin at the same time. However, my body hair is fair and fine so when it grows back it is soft and not very noticeable. If you have darker or thicker hair then microblading may not work so well for you as the regrowing hair may be more obvious and may feel more like stubble. There are many Youtube videos about microblading and I recommend doing some research before trying it on yourself.

For Men
Men have the option of growing a beard or designer stubble and thus eliminating the need for facial shaving altogether. If

you choose to shave you can try dry shaving with an electric razor. From what I understand electric razors never give quite as smooth a shave as wet shaving, but may provide the least irritating option. If you wish to wet shave then you will need to find a soap/shaving cream free of reaction causing chemicals and also razors that either have no moisturising strip or one that is free from problem chemicals. Using a microfiber exfoliating glove after shaving can help smooth flaky skin and reduce ingrown hairs. Apply a small amount of refined jojoba oil or a suitable chemical-free moisturiser (see the section on Skincare above) after shaving to soothe your skin and reduce irritation. For hair removal on other parts of your body you can try waxing or laser hair removal. If you are going to try waxing you will need to check that the wax used is free of chemicals you are intolerant to and also any soothing cream that would normally be applied afterwards. The wax used may be low in salicylates and other chemicals, but the soothing cream applied afterwards is likely to be high in them so either take your own cream to put on, or ask for just an ice-pack to soothe the area that has been waxed.

Sanitary Items

Look for sanitary items that are plastic, perfume and chlorine free. For a number of years, every time I started menstruating I would experience itching in the vaginal area. I thought I was getting thrush every time I got my period which I also thought was strange because it only seemed to occur at that time. I then realised that it wasn't thrush, but that I was reacting to the chemicals in the sanitary pads I was using. I changed to organic cotton sanitary pads and had no further itching issues. I use the Natracare brand and also washable cloth menstrual pads. The Fed-Up website also lists some options (see Recommended Products – Personal Care).

Make-up

I found it very challenging to find make-up that I could use. Not only do I react to nearly all the common ingredients, but my skin is also extremely sensitive and prone to dryness. Andrea Rose produces a range of salicylate and fragrance-free cosmetics as does Cleure. The Fed-Up website also lists options which others have found suitable (see Recommended Products – Personal Care and Make-up).

I personally use mineral make-up products from Immersion cosmetics. Most of the Immersion products are pure minerals free from essential oils. I like the fact that you can order sample packets from this website as I do not wear make-up much so the sample packets give me enough product for a year or so. Mineral make-up powders are very versatile. You can use the foundation powder with a dry brush, or a damp brush, or mix it with a suitable moisturiser to make a tinted moisturiser. You can also make your own concealer or liquid foundation by mixing mineral foundation powder with a small amount of refined jojoba oil or suitable moisturiser to make a paste. Make a thicker paste for concealer and a thinner paste for foundation. Brush mineral powder over the top to set the foundation/concealer after applying it to your face.

Use a slanted brush and small feathery strokes to apply a darker shade of mineral powder to define your brows then smear a little jojoba oil on top to keep brow hairs tidy. Use a wet, fine tipped eye-liner brush with a dark mineral powder to create liquid eye-liner. You can even brush mineral powder blush onto your lips for a lip colour and tap a little moisturiser, shea butter, or jojoba oil over the top for a soft sheen. If you are going to use powder mineral make-up I would advise investing in some good quality make-up brushes to give a flattering finish and keep irritation to your skin to a minimum.

Quick Tip: If you wash your make-up brushes with a mild chemical-free shampoo and then also use conditioner on them the bristles remain soft and are less irritating for sensitive skin.

Nail Care
Buff Your Nails
Nail polish is very high in toxic chemicals. Even if you use a lower chemical version you still have the problem of how to remove it as nail polish remover is also high in chemicals. An alternative is to buff your nails. This does not colour them but it does give them a nice shine that lasts for a few days. Nail buffing blocks are inexpensive and readily available from chemists and department stores. I make a detox/pamper session out of buffing my nails once a week. I fill a large stainless steel bowl with hot water, add 1-2 tablespoons of both Epsom salts (magnesium sulphate) and baking soda, soak my hands then soak my feet while I push back the cuticles on the nails on my hands and buff them. Once I've finished my hands I dry off my feet, push back the cuticles on my toenails and then buff them. Buffing also increases the circulation to your nails, strengthening them and improving their health.

Food Handling and Storage

Glove Up
It took me a while to get used to doing this (and to do it without feeling self-conscious), but it is a wise idea to wear safe kitchen gloves when preparing food. Skin does absorb at least some of what it is exposed to, and many of us experience reactions when our skin comes into contact with chemicals we are sensitive to. You can reduce your exposure by wearing gloves when preparing food, even your own 'safe' food, but definitely any food you prepare for others. When your wear

gloves you wash your hands less often and since it is difficult to find a soap/cleansing product that is safely free of problematic ingredients then the less our skin comes into contact with soap the better. Wearing gloves also reduces the drying effects of water and washing for those of us with eczema on our hands, or sensitive dry skin.

Use Glass or Stainless Steel Storage
Plastic is largely made from petrochemicals and can contain unsafe ingredients like dyes, pthalates and chemical estrogens. To avoid your food being contaminated with extra problematic chemicals it is best to use glass or stainless steel drink bottles and food storage containers. This is particularly important if the food you are storing is hot, or acidic, or contains fats as these types of foods and liquids are even more likely to leach chemicals from a plastic container. Be aware that aluminium drink bottles, as well as being made of potentially toxic aluminium, are also often lined with plastic.

Use Chemical-Free Cookware
The least toxic materials for cookware are heavy metal-free ceramic, enamel and glass. Cast iron cookware is also a good option, but iron does leach into food cooked in it. A little iron can be a healthy, but excess iron is toxic and pro-oxidant. More iron leaches from new cast iron cookware and into acidic foods or foods cooked for long periods. I use cast iron fry-pans. I have found if you season them when you first get them, wash them as soon as you are finished cooking with hot water only (no detergent) and dry them as soon as possible they do not rust and maintain a sealed cooking surface. Be aware that factory/pre-seasoned cast iron pans are usually made by coating the pan in a soy-based oil and then heating it to a high heat so there may be soy, sulphur, glutamate or toxic fat issues. I prefer to season my own to be safe. Copper cookware releases copper into food cooked in it and usually contains nickel which is a toxic heavy metal and can be

allergenic. Stainless steel cookware is made from a metal alloy consisting of mainly iron and chromium, but may also contain nickel along with copper and molybdenum. Stainless steel is a passable option, but not the best. I have read that if a magnet sticks to your stainless-steel cookware, it is likely to be made from mainly non-toxic metals such as iron.

Definitely avoid using any kind of non-stick or aluminium cookware. Most non-stick cookware contains perfluorooctanoic acid (PFOA), especially the brands Teflon, Silverstone, T-Fal, Duracote, Excalibur and Xylon. PFOA gets into your bloodstream, is a xenoestrogen, and may cause flu-like symptoms, cancer, high cholesterol, thyroid disease and reduced fertility. Most manufacturers are phasing out the use of PFOA in cookware, but it will still be found in older items, and may still be in use for new ones, so it is best to avoid non-stick cookware altogether. The other issue with non-stick cookware is that most people use plastic utensils with it which is another source of toxic chemicals, however you can use wooden or silicone utensils instead which are less toxic options. Aluminium is a toxic heavy metal and has been linked to cancer and Alzheimer's disease.

Genuine stoneware such as slabs and pots made of soapstone or lead-free clay are non-toxic. However, these are generally heavy, require seasoning and are higher in price. Most cookware labelled granite or stoneware is actually aluminium with a stone-look non-stick coating. Some brands are potentially non-toxic. Ballarini states that the coating on its granite cookware is PFOA, heavy-metal and nickel free. Theoretically that seems okay, but personally I would stay with safer options instead such as clay-based stoneware, cast iron, ceramic and glass.

Silicone bakeware is another option. The silicone used in bakeware is a synthetic polymer and is generally considered safe and inert, but has not been thoroughly tested at high temperatures. There is potential for chemical leaching and off-gassing when silicone is heated to higher temperatures, especially if it is lower quality silicone which contains fillers. I do use silicone bakeware occasionally because my children and I do not tolerate many fats/oils and you do not have to grease silicone bakeware. I would recommend only using silicone cookware regularly for cooler temperature uses such as chocolate moulds and utensils. You can also get silicone bags for the freezer which would be a less toxic option than plastic.

Ceramic, enamel and glass cookware are the safest options to cook with that are also easy to use and maintain. They are generally very low or toxin free and you can use metal utensils with them. However, be aware that sometimes ceramic glazes and glass can be contaminated with heavy metals such as lead, especially older items and items produced by small scale artisans. Never cook with any ceramic or glass item that is labelled 'for decorative use only'. It is best to avoid cookware with coloured glazes if possible. Older Pyrex cookware was made using a different process to modern Pyrex and is more resilient, so items sourced from
second-hand stores or your grandmother's kitchen might actually last the longest.

Brands which provide non-toxic cookware include: Xtrema ceramic, Le Creuset, Lodge, Mercola Healthy Cookware, The Pampered Chef Stoneware, Chantal, Miriam's Earthen Cookware, Granite Ware, Pyrex and Corningware, Cook on Clay Flameware and Vita Clay. If you like non-stick cookware you could try some from Greenpan, Ecolution, Manpan or Earthpan which are made without PFOA and other toxic chemicals. However, these are all made from coated aluminium and you have to use plastic, silicone or wooden utensils with them.

Buy Meat from a Butcher
The meat packaging used in supermarkets/grocery stores is usually made from petrochemicals and can contain synthetic estrogens. The absorbent pads that are put under the meat can contain sulphites. It is best to buy fresh meat from a reputable butcher with a high turnover of stock which makes it more likely that the meat is fresh. You can take your own glass or stainless steel containers for the butcher to put the meat into. Alternatively, take the meat out of the bags that the butcher put it in and put it into suitable containers as soon as you get home. Buying meat from a butcher also means that you can ask questions about the source, freshness and additives (if any) in the meat.

Cleaning

Modern chemical cleaning products are one of the greatest sources of pollution in our homes, air, clothing and water. Fortunately, there are alternatives that are not only chemical-free, but can also save you time and money. I have listed some options for chemical-free cleaning below. However, my cleaning agent of choice is good quality microfibre cloths. I use Enjo microfibre cloths and I love them. Using microfibre cloths allows me to clean faster, with less effort and more effectively than any other cleaning product I am aware of. Surfaces are left with a long-lasting shine and no residue. You can also clean with cold water which is faster and cheaper - no more lugging round buckets of hot water. Good quality microfibre cloths cost quite a lot up front, but over time save you money as you don't need to buy any other cleaning products for 2-3 years. It is worth paying for quality too as I have tried several cheaper brands and have found that they do not perform as well, or last as long.

Chemical-Free Cleaning Options

Clothes Washing Powder
You can use a fragrance/essential oil free washing detergent. For a totally safe and inexpensive option you can use plain baking soda/sodium bicarbonate as a washing powder. Add about one cup to a full load. I have used this and found that it cleaned the clothes just as effectively as anything else.

Quick Tip: here in New Zealand the cheapest way to buy baking soda is to get it in bulk from a farming supplies store such as PGG Wrightson, or a bulk grocery retailer such as Binn Inn or Bulk Barn (sorry, I'm not sure if this is the case for other countries).

Smelly Shoes
Sprinkle baking soda inside the shoes, leave overnight then shake out the excess.

Carpets
To refresh carpet sprinkle it with sodium bicarbonate, leave it for at least 30 minutes then vacuum as normal. For general stains and marks dab with a cloth dampened with soapy water or use a specifically designed microfiber cloth such as the Enjo Plusline range which I use and recommend.

Polishing Silver and Stainless-Steel
Put a piece of aluminium foil in the bottom of a clean sink. Put your silver or stainless-steel items on top, sprinkle baking soda generously all over them and then pour warm/hot water over the items to cover them. Let the items soak for 10-30 minutes, rub gently with a soft cloth then rinse and dry thoroughly. For heavily tarnished items you may need to repeat this process one or two times.

Dusting
Household dust contains multiple chemical contaminants

from the air, treated carpets, degrading foam in furniture and plastics in electrical appliances. It is important to dust regularly, especially if you have children as they tend to play near dusty surfaces and put their hands near their mouth, nose and eyes more often. To dust effectively, use a damp cloth and then dry off surfaces with a dry cloth afterwards. Dry dusting just moves the dust around unless you use a quality microfibre cloth. I used to avoid dusting because I found wet dusting to be quite a big job with wetting cloths, rinsing cloths and drying off. When I purchased an Enjo dusting cloth I began to dust much more often because it is as effective dry as wet cloth dusting, but much faster. It is also one of the most effective ways to dust things like books and painting canvases which cannot be wet dusted. Remember to wet mop non-carpeted floors regularly too as they also accumulate dust quickly. A microfibre mop is the quickest, easiest way to do this

Clearing the Air
Chemicals from furniture, fragrances, cleaning agents, plastics and electric appliances can build up inside closed indoor spaces. If the outdoor air quality is alright, then open windows and doors to air out your indoor spaces as often as possible. Use pot plants inside and plant trees and shrubs outside to help clear toxins and chemicals out of the air. If you own your own home put an exterior venting fan in the bathroom and kitchen to expel damp air, fragrances used by other members of the household, and chemicals from cooking food and oils, especially if you have people in your house who cook foods that you are intolerant to. It would also be wise to think about investing in an air filtration system. We have an HRV system in our home here in New Zealand and find it very effective. It filters the air of dust particles, spores, pollen and bacteria, and dries out the house which not only makes condensation on windows almost non-existent, but also prevents the growth of toxic moulds.

Remember to clean vent filters frequently, including those in heat pumps and kitchen range hoods. Dust contains many chemical contaminants and clogs up the filter preventing it from working as effectively. If you find cleaning greasy range hood filter pads a hassle, then invest in an Enjo kitchen microfibre glove and drying cloth because they effectively clean the filter pads with COLD water in minutes.

Another way to clear the air is to use odour and chemical absorbing products. I haven't personally used these, but I have seen independent recommendations for the No Odor/Smelleze brand (see Appendix Recommended Products for more information). Using odour and chemical remover pouches would be a cheaper option than installing a whole house filter system and they would also be very handy to take with you when you are travelling.

Treating Day to Day Illness

When you get ill and experience chemical sensitivities your medication options are severely limited. Natural remedies are often high in salicylates, and most pain relief medications cause issues for people with salicylate and histamine intolerance. However, there are still a range of things you can use to treat day to day illnesses and accidents. Fed Up by Sue Dengate has an informative chapter on acceptable medications, and I have also listed a few suitable remedies here.

Calming a Chemical Reaction
The following things should help to calm an especially strong reaction, for example if you have been out to dinner or exposed to a lot of fragrance:

- Drink plenty of clean water to help flush out your detoxification organs (liver and kidneys) and your digestive system and bowel

- Take Iodine: take 1-2 drops of an ionic iodine solution

- Have an epsom salts soak: put 1-2 tablespoons of Epsom salts in a footbath or 1-2 cups in a bath and soak for 10-15 minutes. Alternatively, you can apply epsom salts solution or lotion to your skin.

- Go for a walk in the park: moderate, enjoyable exercise helps relieve physical and emotional stress, stimulate your detoxification systems, and increase oxygen intake decreasing inflammation. Exercise outside around trees or open water is most effective and beneficial.

- Take a magnesium supplement: if you have a magnesium supplement that you tolerate then you can try taking an extra dose

- Take some anti-histamine medication: it is advisable to use anti-histamines as an emergency medication only

- Take some sodium bicarbonate/potassium bicarbonate: add sodium or potassium bicarbonate to a footbath or bath (I sometimes use both Epsom salts and sodium bicarbonate in my footbath for extra detoxing), or mix a ½ teaspoonful into a glass of water and sip. Taking the sodium bicarbonate in a glass of water does not taste very nice, but I find it works well. Sodium/potassium bicarbonate can assist in re-establishing the acid/base balance when your body's own bicarbonate reserves are depleted as a result of metabolic acidosis caused by adverse reactions to food or other environmental exposures. However, please read the following information before taking baking soda internally, and take it only when necessary. It is best to take sodium/potassium bicarbonate at least one hour before or after eating a meal as it lowers the acidity of your stomach reducing digestion, especially of proteins.

PLEASE READ THIS BEFORE TAKING BAKING SODA
Baking soda is SODIUM bicarbonate.
Avoid taking it if you are on a low-sodium diet, or if you are pregnant or breastfeeding.

Avoid taking significant amounts especially for weeks at a time unless under the supervision of a trained health professional.

Sodium bicarbonate inhibits folic acid absorption so you may wish to take a folic acid supplement if you are taking significant amounts of baking soda.

High sodium intake can cause low calcium levels as your kidneys excrete calcium with sodium

If you are taking any prescription medications consult your doctor before taking sodium bicarbonate in case it interferes with your medication.

If you have heart disease, liver disease, kidney disease or high blood pressure consult your doctor before taking baking soda. Avoid giving baking soda to children under five.

If you eat a high calcium/dairy-rich diet or take calcium supplements or calcium-based antacids such as calcium carbonate (e.g. Tums), then be aware that taking significant amounts of sodium bicarbonate can cause milk-alkali syndrome resulting in metastatic calcification, kidney stones and kidney failure.

Taking large amounts of baking soda may cause metabolic alkalosis, or edema, or hypertension due to sodium overload. Stop taking it if you experience nausea, muscle weakness, confusion, swelling of the feet or ankles, black tar-like stools, muscle twitches or tremors, or numbness or tingling in the face or extremities.

Colds
Rest as much as possible and drink plenty of warm fluids (soup, warm/hot water). Take probiotics, zinc, iodine, selenium and vitamin C (see Step 5 – Core Supplementation for information on suitable supplements). Iodine is anti-bacterial and anti-viral and a liquid solution can be put in a spray bottle and used to disinfect the skin of humans and animals as well as the air, furniture and household surfaces. Iodine has been shown to kill most bacteria within 15-30 seconds of contact.

To loosen blocked sinuses put some steaming hot water into a glass or stainless-steel bowl, make a tent over your head with a towel and breathe in the vapours (having a bath or shower also helps clear blocked sinuses). Alternatively, you can sniff up warm salt water. If your child gets earache use the steam measures just mentioned to clear sinus blockages, give them frequent small doses of colloidal silver and put a warm pad on their ear to help relieve pain. Elevating the end of the bed also helps relieve the symptoms of a cold and earache when sleeping. You can do this by putting thick books or bricks under the two legs at the head of the bed.

There is a traditional remedy for colds and flu that uses baking soda (see note above before taking baking soda internally). I haven't tried it myself, but here are the recommended doses if you want to try it:

Day 1: take 6 doses of a ½ teaspoon of baking soda in a glass of warm or room temperature water at about 2 hourly intervals
Day 2: take 4 doses of a ½ teaspoon of baking soda in a glass of warm or room temperature water at about 2 hourly intervals
Day 3: take 2 doses of a ½ teaspoon of baking soda in a glass of warm or room temperature water – one in the morning and one in the evening. From day 4 onwards take a ½ teaspoon of baking soda in water each morning until the cold/flu symptoms are completely gone.

Sore throat: gargle warm salt water and/or one drop of iodine in warm water. Take probiotics and/or colloidal silver. Take probiotics and colloidal silver several hours apart or the colloidal silver may kill off some of the probiotics. I am wary of taking colloidal silver because it is a metal. It does seem to help so I use it, but only for bacterial illnesses and only until symptoms clear.

Coughs: the best thing I have found to calm a cough is to sip whiskey or vodka mixed with a little warm water, but of course this can't be given to children. I give my children probiotics and colloidal silver to help treat the infection causing the cough. It also helps to keep the bedroom slightly warm at night. Saffron is a traditional remedy for coughs. Make a tea by infusing a few saffron threads in hot water. Once the water has cooled to warm, remove the threads and gargle the saffron tea.

Cuts and Sores
Wash or soak gently with warm water and an appropriate soap. Keep them clean and dry. You can apply colloidal silver or iodine (see colds above) to help prevent or treat infection and refined jojoba oil to help skin heal.

Fungal Infections
For fungal infections on your toenails try applying a mix of

lemon and potato juice 2-3 times a day. This may require several weeks of daily application. Potatoes have anti-fungal and anti-viral properties. The juice is best applied as fresh as possible. Lemons have a low to moderate level of salicylates. They have anti-fungal and anti-bacterial properties. If you paint the lemon juice onto the nail, then only a very small amount will be absorbed via the surrounding skin. Note that fungal infections are infectious so wash your hands thoroughly after touching any infected area.

If you can tolerate coconut oil, then it also has anti-fungal properties. Again, regular application is key to effectiveness. Apply it 2-3 times a day until the symptoms clear. Coconut oil has also been shown to help clear yeast infections.

Insect Bites
Apply a paste of baking soda and water to the bite to relieve itching. Bee stings are acidic so put baking soda on them which is an alkali. Wasp stings are alkaline so you can treat them by putting vinegar on them.

Pain
Use warm pads or ice packs – whichever gives the best relief. Only ice an inflamed area for a few minutes at a time.

Pimples
Dab colloidal silver on the pimple as it is anti-bacterial. Iodine is also anti-bacterial, but many people find iodine actually makes their acne worse. This may however be due to a detox reaction that settles with prolonged use. Saffron is apparently helpful – you could try infusing a couple of threads in water or refined jojoba oil and dabbing it on the spot. I find that my acne is caused by stress, salicylates and also fragrances, especially cheap ones like supermarket body sprays. Reducing inflammation will reduce the severity and pain of pimples.

Stomach Bug/Food Poisoning/Diarrhoea
I find that colloidal silver and probiotics help clear stomach issues relatively quickly. Take them several hours apart as per the instructions for a sore throat above.

Sunburn
Add ½ cup of baking soda to a lukewarm bath and soak for 10-15minutes. When you get out try and let the baking soda dry on your skin rather than towelling it off. You can also make a compress by soaking a towel in a solution of baking soda and cool water, wringing out the excess water then placing the towel on the sunburnt area.

Warts
Warts are caused by a virus. Please note that because of this they are infectious so wash your hands thoroughly after touching warts. You can have them burnt off with dry ice (carbon dioxide) by a doctor. Potatoes have anti-viral properties. A possible treatment for warts is to apply potato juice to the wart 3 times a day. Use juice that is as fresh as possible. You may need to continue this treatment for several weeks to see results. Banana peel is another possible treatment. Scrape the white flesh off the inside of a piece of banana peel and then apply the small piece of exposed inner peel to the wart and cover it with a plaster. Apply fresh peel twice a day. Coconut oil also has anti-viral properties, and may be used to treat warts if you can tolerate it. Apply it to the wart as per potato juice.

Odd Extras

Relax in Nature
The best leisure activities are those that involve activity

outside amongst nature. Trees and plants help to clear some chemicals from the air and produce oxygen which also helps our detoxification systems work more effectively. Swimming pools, shopping malls and roadsides contain concentrations of chemicals and are best avoided. Going for a walk or cycle ride through gardens, forests or beaches, or going skiing, are leisure activities that do not involve exposure to a lot of chemicals.

Avoid Public Toilets
Public toilets that are cleaned regularly such as those in busy shopping malls have high concentrations of cleaning chemicals on the basins and toilets, and in the air. Think like a child and try and go to the toilet at home before you go out. If you do have to use a public bathroom either carry your own hand-wash or just rub your hands vigorously under hot water to wash them (bacteria is removed by friction) and then dry them thoroughly in an air-dryer (bacteria needs moisture to survive and grow).

Buy Groceries Online
I find that supermarkets are high in chemical levels especially the cleaning, personal care and spice/baking aisles. Added into that is the fragrances worn by the people shopping and working there. For super-responders like me it is a bit of a minefield. You can avoid this by ordering your groceries online. The down side with buying groceries online is that you cannot read ingredient labels, so it is only suitable for buying products you have already identified to be safe.

Let Someone Else Refuel the Car
Petrochemicals can cause a reaction or worsen other chemical sensitivities. If possible, get someone else to put petrol/diesel in your vehicle and lawnmower. Liquid petroleum gas (LPG) may also cause problems and is best avoided.

Use Electric Cookers Rather Than Gas if Possible
We stayed at a house once that had a gas cooker. I hadn't been exposed to one since my chemical sensitivities had become inflamed, but when I started cooking on it my eczema started to flare up significantly and I experienced headaches and nausea.

Grow Safe Greenery
Living plants clear the air of chemicals and give off cleansing oxygen so grow them inside and out, but avoid plants with strong scents such as fragrant flowers and pungent herbs. Avoid using chemical sprays in your garden. Remove weeds manually, and use non-chemical options for bug control such as companion planting and putting coffee grounds or egg shells around plants to deter slugs and snails. If you live somewhere with limited outdoor space, then consider growing a green 'wall' i.e., grow plants vertically.

Buy Natural Rubber or Leather Footwear
Jandals/thongs/flip-flops are often made of foam and resin containing phenols and aldehydes, both of which can be a problem for those of us with chemical sensitivities. Buy natural leather or rubber footwear instead. See Recommended Products in the Appendix for some options.

Leave Your Shoes at the Door
Wearing shoes inside that you have been walking around in outside brings many pollutants into your home for example herbicide/pesticide sprays used in public gardens and parks and petrochemical residues. Put a shoe rack by the front door and teach your children to take off their shoes and put them on the rack as soon as they come inside. Invest in some comfortable, attractive slippers to wear around the house.

Support Companies that have Publicly Committed to going PBDE-free

Acer, Apple, Eizo Nanao, LG Electronics, Lenovo, Matsushita, Microsoft, Nokia, Phillips, Samsung, Sharp, Sony-Ericsson, and Toshiba have publically committed to removing PBDE chemicals from their electrical appliances.

Step 5: Add Effective Supplements

(Please note, the information in this chapter regarding supplements was current as at September 2015. Manufacturers change the ingredients in their products from time to time so it is always wise to re-check ingredient listings, which sometimes may require contacting the manufacturer, before taking any supplements.)

Do I Need to take Nutritional Supplements?

The answer to this varies from person to person. You may need to take supplements initially to help promote healing in your body. Once significant healing has taken place then you will probably be able to reduce the number and amount of supplements you take. Or, if your intolerance is not too severe, then simply putting into place the actions outlined in Step One to Four of this book may be enough to keep you largely symptom free and able to eat a significant number of different foods.

Most people in modern westernised societies are mineral deficient due to a high intake of processed foods and sugar. In addition, the soil in most parts of the world now contains far fewer minerals than it did in the past meaning that the plants grown in that soil absorb, and consequently contain, low levels of minerals. Anyone with digestive health issues, which is likely to be all of us with food and chemical intolerances, will probably poorly absorb nutrients from the food they are eating and have lower levels of the vitamins produced by the gut such as vitamin K and B vitamins. This means that most of you reading this book are likely to have low levels of many vitamins and minerals even without considering the fact that your diet is very limited.

My experience of supplements has been a long, costly one of trial and often painful error. I have arrived at the point now where I believe it is best for me to focus on self-care treatments such as rest, exercise and enjoyment. I take the core supplements listed below but not much beyond that as I have experienced numerous severe adverse reactions to supplements. I also carry round some mother-guilt from having given my children supplements which I thought would be helpful, only to have them react to them with pain and discomfort. Supplements can be very helpful, but definitely proceed with caution when it comes to taking them. Below are some points to consider before taking any nutritional supplements.

Choose Supplements Carefully
Many vitamin/mineral supplements contain flavourings, colourings or other chemicals you may react to and some trace ingredients are not listed so you may have to contact the manufacturer to find out exactly every ingredient that is in a product. Colourings and flavourings are fairly obvious additives to avoid, but others may not be so clear. Magnesium stearate seems to be a problem for me. It is a filler/flow agent that can be contaminated with pesticides and xenoestrogens and may have a detrimental effect on your immune and digestive systems. Another filler to be aware of is coconut derived MCT oil which is often listed as 'triglicerides'. Cellulose capsules are made from plant material so it is best to buy liquid supplements, or pour the contents of the capsule onto food or into water and discard the capsule. Sometimes cellulose is a filler as well though. Ingredients with 'citrate' at the end are usually corn based.

Supplements that contain multiple nutrients are also often problematic as there are often one or two things in the mix which may cause issues. Beware of boron. It is often found in calcium, vitamin D and multi-mineral supplements (pears and apples are also high in boron). Boron causes excretion of vitamin B2 and may inhibit detoxification. I find that it is best to opt for single nutrient supplements with no or few fillers and definitely no flavourings or colourings. Vegetable capsules are a better option than tablets. Capsules generally have fewer additives and it is also easier to open the capsule for smaller doses.

Another thing to be aware of is that nutritional supplements are usually highly concentrated so while the physical amount of a problematic substance may be very small, it is likely to have a magnified impact. Some of my most severe reactions have been to very small amounts of nutritional supplements.

Things to Avoid for Specific Chemical Intolerances

General
Chromium: excess chromium can cause your body to excrete sulphate through the kidneys rather than utilising it in your body. It is critical that those of us with chemical intolerances absorb and retain all the sulphate we can

Histamine Intolerance
If you have a histamine intolerance it is recommended that you avoid the following supplements because they are histamine liberators:
- Folic acid
- Iodine, potassium iodide, potassium iodate

Sulphur Intolerance
If you have a sulphur intolerance the following things may cause issues for you:

- Maltodextrin (often in enzymes and probiotics)
- Herbal tinctures: most herbal tinctures are made using a corn based alcohol
- Gelatin capsules: the processing of gelatin usually includes sulphites
- ALA (Alpha Lipoic Acid): this is commonly used for chelation purposes to cleanse your body of heavy metals. If you are sulphur-sensitive, you may only tolerate small amounts of ALA, so start low just in case.
- Bromelain and papain (use enzymes derived from animals instead of these)
- Chlorella
- Cysteine
- Methionine (converts down into cysteine)
- Dairy source acidophilus
- DMSO
- Extracts of high sulphur foods
- Glutathione
- NAC
- MSM
- Turmeric

Glutamate Intolerance

If you have a glutamate intolerance the following things may cause issues for you:
- Glutamine (glutamic acid): converts to glutamate in your brain. This is mainly prescribed to heal intestinal damage. I tried it and had a severe reaction.
- Algae/seaweed based supplements
- Anything that contains corn or soy or ingredients derived from corn and soy

You May Get Worse While Getting Better

Be aware before you begin that sometimes taking supplements that help can initially provoke symptoms of chemical/food intolerance. This can make it difficult to know whether something is helping or just causing a reaction. The only way to really tell if this is the case, is time. I found that with myself and my children when a supplement caused our food intolerance symptoms to become worse that it would take about 2-3 weeks to hit a turning point where the reaction symptoms would begin to go away. Usually, you can also see some difference i.e., there might be some positive responses as well as negative ones or the reaction symptoms might be slightly different to normal.

Go Slow

We all want to get better quickly, but unfortunately when you are dealing with chemical intolerances, especially if you are particularly sensitive like myself and my children, you have to proceed very slowly with a recovery plan. Start with very small doses of one supplement and only increase it when it does not appear to cause any negative symptoms. Increase it slowly. Only introduce another supplement once you have achieved a moderate to full dose of the previous one and/or you have worked out what dose is right for you. Establish one supplement at a time. This gives your body time to adjust, and enables you to see clearly the effect each supplement is having.

This is a long slow process. It can be frustratingly slow at times especially in the beginning, but I believe this is the best way to get long lasting results. It also saves you money sometimes as you can clearly see if a particular supplement is right for you or not, or whether you need to any further supplements at all. We are all different. For some of you just increasing your sulphate intake may be enough to reduce your symptoms to a level you are comfortable with. For others, you may find two or three of the core supplements are enough, or that taking all of the supplements listed gives you the best result.

More Is Not Necessarily Better
With some supplements a little is helpful, but more may not give any better results than a smaller dose, or may even be harmful. When I outline the specific supplements below I note whether excessive amounts may have a negative effect. For some supplements, such as probiotics and enzymes in particular, it is matter of trial and error to find your personal equilibrium i.e., how much gives you the maximum benefit before more than that does not give any further improvements or starts to give you adverse results.

I have begun this list of supplements with four core supplements. I call these core supplements because they will assist with all the intolerances covered in this book: histamine, sulphur, glutamate and salicylate sensitivity. They are also the most commonly recommended, and the ones that significant numbers of people have found helpful.

The Core Supplements
Sulphate (including zinc and magnesium)
Probiotics
Vitamin D
Digestive Enzymes

Core Supplement 1: Sulphate (Magnesium and Zinc Sulphate)
It is thought that most phenol, chemical and sulphur intolerance is caused by a poorly functioning sulphation detoxification pathway. This pathway involves the enzyme Phenol Sulphur-tranferase (PST) combining with sulphate to transport chemical compounds out of your body. PST detoxifies leftover hormones and a wide variety of toxic molecules, such as phenols and amines that are produced in the body and in the gut by bacteria, yeast, and other fungi, as well as food dyes and chemicals. The primary reason this

sulphation process does not work efficiently is usually because a person has low or no ability to convert compounds to sulphate and consequently has very low blood levels of sulphate and insufficient sulphate to effectively process phenolic compounds. Poor sulphation can also be caused by low levels of the PST enzyme. One way to correct this is to provide the body with more sulphate. PST enzymes need sulphur to be formed and they need sulphate to bind to toxic substances to solubilise them so that the kidneys can remove them. Sulphates are also anti-histamines, and are needed to maintain the integrity of the gut wall, and for the release of pepsin, stomach acid and digestive enzymes.

The reasons I start with a sulphate supplement are:
1. It helps detoxify your body

2. If it helps then it is a good indication that your chemical intolerance symptoms are caused by this fault in your detoxification pathways and it is nice to have some idea of what causes the problem.

3. It is the cheapest supplement and may be all that you need

The easiest and most inexpensive way to take sulphate is to use magnesium sulphate in the form of Epsom salts. You can buy Epsom salts at most supermarkets and chemists. You take this form of sulphate via the skin (transdermally) by adding the Epsom salts to a bath or footbath, or by putting a solution of them on your skin. I had tried having Epsom salts footbaths in the past, but always had reaction symptoms afterwards and so I thought that I reacted to them and avoided exposing myself to any more. I then read that it is common to have a reaction at first so I started putting a solution on my skin instead. I began with one drop per day of a solution of one tablespoon water to one teaspoon Epsom salts. I did have minor reaction symptoms again, but this time I persisted and began to slowly increase the dose by one drop each day or two. After a while I noticed that I had a small flush of symptoms soon after I put the Epsom salt solution on my skin and then the symptoms would fade with no further problems. When I got to a moderate sized dose, I began to have very little reaction at all.

I started off taking magnesium sulphate in the form of Epsom salts. However, as I started increasing the dose, I found that I was feeling hot and flushed quite a lot. Someone told me that magnesium can have a heating effect on the body. To see if this was what was causing the problem, I started using zinc sulphate instead. The feelings of being hot and flushed stopped as soon as I swapped to the zinc sulphate. Most people are fine with the magnesium sulphate, but be aware that it may cause some issues, and if it does you may want to try another form of sulphate. However, I am also wary of taking too much zinc because it can lead to the creation of more histamine (see the section on zinc below). I now take a balance of transdermal doses of zinc sulphate and magnesium sulphate.

Taking sulphate in the form of magnesium sulphate and zinc sulphate also provides you with two other beneficial minerals without having to take extra supplements. Additionally, it provides them in a readily absorbed, non-additive form reducing the risk of reaction to the encapsulating aids used in tablets and capsules. People with digestive health issues usually do not absorb magnesium well from their digestive system. Magnesium and zinc (along with selenium) may help protect glutamate receptors from excessive absorption.

Magnesium
Magnesium is the most important mineral in the human body because it is a co-factor for more than 300 enzymes. It

activates the sulphation detoxification enzyme phenol-sulphotransferase. Your body requires adequate levels of magnesium for digestion, detoxification and to help regulate bowel movements. Excess magnesium is not particularly harmful and you know when you are consuming excessive amounts because it will make you pass frequent, loose stools (taking magnesium is a good way to help clear constipation). When you are stressed, your body uses more magnesium and if you are deficient in magnesium, it will magnify stress reactions. Lack of magnesium can also cause disturbed sleep. Magnesium is required for muscle relaxation which is why signs of deficiency include muscle cramps and facial muscle tics and twitching. Taking magnesium before bed often helps promote good sleep.

Zinc

Zinc is needed for optimum immune function and is involved in wound healing and protein synthesis. Zinc is needed to produce hydrochloric acid (HCL) in your stomach. Zinc must be ingested on a daily basis as your body has no capacity to store it. Be aware that your zinc and copper levels need to be balanced for optimal health. High zinc intake can lead to copper deficiency. If you take a zinc supplement, then I would advise you to get your zinc and copper levels checked regularly to ensure the correct balance is maintained. Also, taking too much zinc may cause your body to start converting the amino acid histidine into histamine.

How to Take Magnesium and Zinc Sulphate

For magnesium sulphate I make up a solution of 1 tablespoon Epsom salts to 3 tablespoons filtered water and store it in a glass dropper bottle. I put drops of this solution onto areas of our body where the skin is thin or absorbent such as feet, shins and forearms and then lightly rub it in. You can also mix this Epsom salts solution with a cream or mix Epsom salts into a lotion. Alternatively, add some Epsom Salts to a footbath or bath.

Use the zinc sulphate that comes in an ionic liquid form. Zinc sulphate can be taken internally, but I apply this transdermally on the skin also. The reason for this is that people with chemical intolerances often have gut damage or dysfunction and do not absorb nutrients well when they are ingested orally.

Core Supplement 2: Probiotics
There is a multitude of scientific evidence demonstrating that consuming probiotic (good) bacteria is significantly beneficial for our overall health and for our immune and digestive systems in particular. There is also considerable scientific evidence demonstrating that taking high dose probiotic supplements can help reduce the intensity of allergies and food and chemical intolerances. In general, probiotic bacteria produce enzymes, amino acids and vitamins. Taking quality probiotic and enzyme supplements can increase the amount of nutrition that you get from food thus reducing the need for other nutrient supplements. Probiotic bacteria clean your intestinal walls, re-establish the balance of intestinal flora and disable harmful organisms without side effects and without causing resistant bacteria to develop. Pathogenic (bad) bacteria, yeast and fungi in your gut produce toxins which put an extra strain on your already low functioning detoxification systems. Increasing the levels of probiotic bacteria in your body helps to reduce the amount and activity of these toxin producing microbes.

Prescriptive strength Lactobacillus and Bifidobacterium have been shown to improve gut-barrier function by increasing tight-junction regulation and reducing inflammation. According to the Salicylate Sensitivity website, research indicates that the probiotic bacteria in our digestive systems play a role in producing sulphate which is needed to detoxify salicylates and other chemicals. Moreover, bacterial imbalance in your digestive system can lead to nutrient deficiencies that can trigger or intensify chemical sensitivities. However, there are some things to be aware of before you start taking a probiotic supplement.

Amines/Histamine
Most probiotic supplements are produced by fermentation and contain amines/histamine. However, some probiotic strains are less problematic than others (see the section below titled Take the Right Strains to find out which). I have a histamine intolerance, but do seem to be able to take certain probiotic supplements without experiencing significant reactionary symptoms. I find the benefits of taking probiotics daily far outweigh any slight reaction to the amines.

Beware of Additives and Fillers
Many probiotics contain maltodextrin which usually contains glutamates and is made from wheat or corn (often genetically modified corn). Probiotic supplements may also contain other corn based free-flow agents not listed as an ingredient. Look for a product that specifically states it is free of corn and wheat. Be aware that some trace additives are not mentioned in the ingredients listing because companies are not required to list ingredients if they are below a certain percentage. However, the small amount may be enough to cause a reaction for us super-responders. If you are extremely sensitive, then it is best to contact the manufacturer to find out everything that is in the product.

Take Enough, but Start with a Very Low Dose
Just eating yogurt on a daily basis will not provide enough probiotic bacteria to make much of an impact (yogurt also contains only the strains of probiotic bacteria that are potentially inflammatory). For prevention and maintenance take ten to fifteen billion CFU (colony forming units) per day.

To treat an illness or for more intensive healing take 20-40 billion CFU per day.

I had been taking one capsule of quality probiotics every day for years without seeing much impact either positively or negatively. I then read that a therapeutic dose of probiotics which was needed for the health issues I was experiencing was 3-4 times the dose I had been taking. When I began to increase the dose of probiotics I was taking to two capsules then three capsules a day, my skin became very inflamed and sensitive and I developed large cystic acne lesions. It took 2-3 weeks after each increase for the skin sensitivity and acne to subside. The pattern was the same for my daughter. When I first started giving her a pinch of probiotic powder each day her food intolerance behavioural issues increased for 2-3 weeks and then calmed down again. I increased my daughter's dosage much more slowly so the adverse reaction was not too uncomfortable.

Not Everyone Can Take Probiotic Supplements
It appears that probiotic supplements are not tolerated at all by some people. If you have thyroid disease, Small Intestinal Bacterial Overgrowth (SIBO) or short-bowel syndrome then you should seek professional advice before taking a probiotic supplement. My son does not seem to tolerate probiotic supplements. I have tried numerous different probiotic products with him and he hasn't been able to tolerate even minute amounts of any of them. Even after months of giving him the smallest pinch he still reacts. It never 'settles'. Probiotic supplements generally make him agitated and clumsy like he's busting to go to the toilet all the time. They also seem to give him increased mucus.

Take the Right Strains
Some common strains of probiotic bacteria are potentially harmful or aggravating for people with certain health issues

and some of these strains are also potentially inflammatory for everyone. There is some evidence that the probiotic strains Lactobacillus and Bifidobacterium may aggravate autoimmune thyroid disease. These strains have also been shown to cause eosinophilic syndrome which is a condition in which the eosiniophils, a type of white blood cell essential to the immune system, become elevated and damage the cardiovascular system, nervous system or bone marrow. Lactobacilli based probiotics may also cause increased lactic acid production in the gut which may be a problem, particularly for children and those with Small Intestinal Bacterial Overgrowth (SIBO) or short-bowel syndrome, or for those who have had a jejunoileal bypass or bowel resection.

Here are the strains that may be beneficial in terms of reducing histamine and inflammation

- *L. Paracasei* – may reverse gut permeability (leaky gut) and internal hypersensitivity
- *L. Rhamnosus* – may prevent harmful bacteria from adhering to your intestinal tract. It also down-regulates allergy and histamine receptors and enhances the activity of anti-inflammatory agents.
- *Lactobacillus helveticus* - may prevent harmful bacteria from adhering to your intestinal tract
- *Bifidobacterium infantis*
- *Bifidobacterium longum*
- *Lactobacillus plantarum* – lowers/inhibits biogenic amines such as tyramine and histamine
- *Lactobacillus reuteri* – may release a histamine that lowers inflammation
- *Bacillus subtilis* – studies have shown this to reduce pro-inflammatory cytokines and increase anti-inflammatory cytokines
- Some soil-based organisms

Neutral Strains
- *Lactobacillus acidophilus* - The DDS-1 Lactobacilli acidophilus strain has been investigated extensively and has been shown to be very stable. It produces a natural antibiotic and inhibits the growth of 23 toxin-producing microorganisms. It also produces folic acid, vitamin B-12 and enzymes which digest protein, fat and lactase. Lastly, it produces hydrogen peroxide to fight adverse bacterial and yeast overgrowth and decreases intestinal inflammation.
- *Lactobacillus lactis*

Strains that May Cause Inflammation/Raise Histamine
- *Lactobacillus casei*
- *Lactobacillus Bulgaricus*

If you have autoimmune thyroid disease, SIBO, short-bowel syndrome or have had a jejunoileal bypass or bowel resection then you may be better to try a probiotic supplement containing soil-based organisms. The *Seeking Health Probiota Infant* probiotic may also be suitable as it contains mainly anti-inflammatory or neutral strains of bacteria and the product description states that it contains only Lactobacillus strains that do not produce difficult to process lactic acid. However, the *Probiota Infant* probiotic contains inulin from chicory root which is very high in salicylates. My daughter and I had very strong salicylate reactions to this product. *Custom Probiotics* also produce a *D-Lactate Free Probiotic Powder* with mainly beneficial bacteria strains.

For children it is preferable to use a low-lactic acid producing probiotic such as soil-based organisms, or a product that states it is low lactic acid producing.

Refrigerated or Shelf-stable - Which is Best?
There is much debate about whether refrigerated or shelf-

stable probiotics are best and there are good arguments on either side. Some argue that if a probiotic must be refrigerated then it its ability to survive in the warm, acidic environment of your stomach is questionable. These people prefer shelf-stable strains which can withstand stomach acid and survive intact to inoculate your upper and lower intestines. Whichever type you choose, it is important to keep the probiotics as dry as possible because moisture will cause them to activate in the container. Take probiotics as soon as you get them out of the container. It is best not to add them to a smoothie and then take it to work to drink for example. Keep the packet of moisture absorbing material in the container and keep the lid of the container securely closed. Generally, it is best practice to keep probiotics refrigerated after the container has been opened whether they are shelf-stable or not.

Recommended Probiotics
I have yet to find a probiotic product that has a perfect combination of anti-inflammatory strains and no other ingredients that contain either wheat, dairy, corn or salicylates. The best I know of at this point are:

Naturopathica GastroHealth
This is recommended by many people on the Failsafe diet. It contains only anti-inflammatory L. Rhamnosus, Lactobacillus helveticus, Bifidobacterium longum and Saccharomyces cerevisiae (boulardii) which is a strain of yeast that has been shown to help restore the natural flora in the large and small intestine and inhibit pathogens. Research has shown that Saccharomyces cerevisiae (boulardii) is effective in treating gastroenteritis which some researchers have linked to high-histamine/mast cell issues. Saccharomyces cerevisiae does contain some natural (bound) glutamic acid which may cause problems for those of us who are sensitive to glutamates.

I have enquired, but haven't been able to find out what, if any, prebiotics and fillers are in the *GastroHealth* probiotic products. I assume it is Failsafe as it has been taken successfully by those connected with the *Fed-Up* website. However, sometimes prebiotics are made from legumes which are failsafe, but may not be suitable for those of us with sulphur or histamine issues. I presume the *GastroHealth Daily Probiotic* is not dairy free because there is a separate dairy free product.

Pro-bio by Enzymedica
This probiotic contains mainly anti-inflammatory strains of bacteria and has no fillers or prebiotics. It is just 8 probiotic strains in a cellulose capsule. Enzymedica is a well regarded brand.

Prescript Assist Soil Based Organisms
This product contains bamboo extract as a prebiotic ingredient. Bamboo shoots are low salicylate so I would assume this is too. *Prescript Assist* contains Bacillus subtilis and 28 strains of other beneficial bacteria. I have not identified any ingredients in this probiotic that may be a problem, and it is well researched and highly recommended by many health professionals. It appears to be tolerated well by people with histamine intolerance.

However, when my son and I tried this probiotic, we had problems. It appeared to cause my son significant digestive upset even at very low doses. I also often felt slightly nauseous after taking it on an empty stomach in the morning and it seemed to cause painful bloating which just got worse the more I took. Surprisingly, it also gave my husband significant digestive upset. He only took it for just over a week so this may have passed for him if he persisted taking it. It may have just been an initial adjustment response. I suspect that my son and I had a problem with the fibrous nature of the bamboo prebiotic. My son and I have very sensitive guts and fibre causes us digestive upset. We do better with the *Pro-bio Probiotic* which has no prebiotics.

Dr Clark Royal Flora soil based probiotics
Along with the probiotic organisms this also contains humic/fulvic acids, bilberry leaf, ginger root, milk thistle seed and cilantro leaf making it unsuitable for people with salicylate sensitivity.

Make sure any probiotic supplement you take is from a good quality brand, contains multiple live strains and is free from contamination by dairy, gluten, soy, corn, wheat, egg and nuts.

Core Supplement 3: Vitamin D
Vitamin D is a fat soluble 'vitamin' (it is technically a prohormone - a precursor of a biologically active hormone). Vitamin D has anti-inflammatory properties and plays a role in:
- calcium uptake and utilisation
- fat metabolism
- regulating and normalising immune response
- supporting healthy insulin action and glucose metabolism

Ideally, we should get our vitamin D from sun exposure to our skin, and if you are able to maintain good vitamin D levels by getting adequate safe sun exposure then that is recommended rather than taking a supplement. However, many of us work indoors, or live in climates that do not provide adequate sun exposure, especially in winter, to maintain high enough vitamin D levels. Getting hot in the sun also raises histamine levels. Thus, for many of us. a vitamin D3 supplement is necessary to maintain optimum vitamin D levels.

It is a good idea to take vitamin K2 when you are taking vitamin D3 because they work together to ensure calcium is put where it needs to go in your body. Take them together, in the morning, with a meal containing fat to ensure they are absorbed. If you cannot or do not wish to take a vitamin K2 supplement, then it is best to take vitamin D supplements with a meal high in vitamin K from free-range animal protein and leafy greens.

Magnesium and zinc are also key co-factors for the absorption and utilization of vitamin D. For optimum benefit take between 2,000-5,000 IU of vitamin D3 a day unless you suffer from hyperparathyroid disease in which case do not take more than 1,000 IU a day. Aim to maintain a blood level between 55-80 ng/dl.

Core Supplement 4: Digestive Enzymes
Enzymes are protein molecules and all cells require enzymes to survive and function. They are catalysts which make chemical reactions go faster, but are not changed by the reaction. Enzymes are required for your body to function properly because without enzymes you wouldn't be able to breathe, swallow, drink, eat, or digest your food. It is largely enzymes which break down the food you eat and then control the reactions which direct how the nutrients from your food are utilised by your body. Research has shown that people who have a chronic disease or have low energy levels also have lower enzyme content in their blood, urine, and tissues.

Our enzyme supply or potential is decreased by a number of factors including:
- Poor dietary habits such as excessive intake of processed foods, fat and sugars

- Stress: stress kills and damages cells, resulting in our enzyme-making machinery having to work overtime to help rebuild and replace them.

> Environmental pollution which causes cellular damage requiring ongoing assistance from enzymes just to maintain a healthy immune system.

> Free radical damage: environmental pollution, overly processed fast foods, genetically modified food and microwave cooking can result in free radical damage, which lowers your body's ability to produce enzymes

> Time: time and the process of living uses up and wears out our enzymes

There are a wide range of digestive enzymes available, but I am going to focus on digestive enzymes designed for chemical intolerance.

Digestive Enzymes for Salicylate Sensitivity
I am aware of three digestive enzyme products designed specifically for salicylate and phenol intolerance:
> *NoFenol* by Houston Enzymes
> *Phenol Assist* by Kirkman Labs
> *Phenolgest* by Enzymedica

These digestive enzyme products are similar in many ways, but also have some differing ingredients. Some ingredients may cause issues for some people. *NoFenol* contains a coconut derived filler: MCT oil. *Phenol Assist* contains no additives other than cellulose and water. However, the carrier for some of the enzymes in *Phenol Assist* is maltodextrin which is usually corn derived. It is highly likely that the corn used for this is genetically modified. Maltodextrin is also a histamine release/mast cell degranulation trigger and is likely to contain free glutamic acid (MSG) as well as being problematic for those of us with sulphur intolerance. The amount of maltodextrin per capsule is extremely small though.

Phenolgest is produced by *Enzymedica* which is a quality brand. Their website states that *Enzymedica* does not use ingredients produced using biotechnology, and *Phenolgest* is said to be free from corn which implies that there is no corn-based maltodextrin anywhere in the product. However, be aware that *Phenolgest* contains protease enzymes and the *NoFenol* and *Phenol Assist* do not. Proteases can be more healing, but they are also more likely to cause gut irritation especially if your gut is injured in any way. Proteases can also be a trigger for people with glutamate intolerance. The amount of proteases in *Phenolgest* is low. If you have a very sensitive gut (which is the case for most people with food and chemical intolerances) then either start with a very small amount of *Phenolgest* and build up very slowly, or take a non-protease containing enzyme such as *NoFenol* or *Phenol Assist* for 2-3 months and then switch to *Phenolgest* if you want to. Protease enzymes help to break down protein so they may help you metabolise and absorb more highly beneficial amino acids and B vitamins.

Digestive Enzymes for Histamine Intolerance
Histamine Intolerance (HIT) is often caused by low levels of the enzyme system called Diamine Oxidase (DAO), which breaks down excess histamine. You can purchase DAO enzyme supplements, but they are not commonly recommended by experts on HIT. This is partly because research on their safety and effectiveness is currently limited, and also because they are often made from pork glands and many people react to pork. I have not tried them, but from my research I understand that they work in much the same way as the enzymes for phenol sensitivity in that you take them before eating histamine containing foods to help break down histamine. You can make your own DAO enzyme 'supplement' from pea-sprouts as discussed in Step 3 –

Prioritise Nutrition on page 78.

How to Take Digestive Enzymes
Enzymes need to be in physical contact with an appropriate food or substance to work. If you are taking the enzymes in the cellulose capsule, then you may need to take the capsule 15-20 minutes before eating to allow time for the capsule to dissolve and the enzymes to be released into your digestive system. If you are opening the capsule and taking the enzyme powder mixed with food or water, then you may be able to take it just before eating. However, some people find that even when taking the enzymes without the capsule they need to take it 15-30 minutes before a meal for the enzymes to help. You will need to experiment to find what works best for you. Unfortunately, like most things concerning chemical intolerance there is no quick process, and trial and adjustment is needed to see what works best for your body.

When you first begin taking digestive enzymes you can expect to experience some digestive upset owing to changes in your gut flora. Common symptoms include increased stool frequency, intestinal wind, mild queasiness and sometimes diarrhoea. These symptoms should last only one to two weeks and can be minimised by starting with very low doses.

The general experience of people seems to be that enzyme products for phenol and histamine sensitivities do help, but usually only mildly. You need to take relatively high doses to give a significant impact and this can become expensive. Many people only take them when they are going to have a particularly high phenol/salicylate/histamine meal, for example if they are eating away from home. You may need to try several different brands of enzymes to find the one that works best for you. I have tried two different brands of enzymes designed to help process phenols. They both helped, but I tolerated one far better than the other and when I began taking it the almost constantly inflamed eczema mask that covered my neck and décolleté calmed and cleared. Remember though, that we are all unique and what works best for one person may not work best for another. While we can be guided by the experiences of others, in the end you do need to try things for yourself.

If you do want to try taking enzymes, and to try detoxing or healing with enzymes, then I highly recommend first reading Karen DeFelice's book *Enzymes: Go With Your Gut* (see Recommended Resources in the Appendix for more information).

Notes on Other Supplements
The following nutritional supplements may also be helpful for some people.

Vitamin K
Vitamin K is a fat-soluble vitamin and comes in two forms. Vitamin K1, the predominant circulating form, is found in green leafy vegetables, liver, fish meal and some dietary oils including olive, hemp, canola, soybean and cottonseed oils. Vitamin K2 can be found in chicken egg yolk, butter, cow liver, certain cheeses, and fermented soybean products such as natto, and it is also produced by intestinal bacteria. Many of the recent studies on Vitamin K have found that the K2 form is the most beneficial.

One of the main roles of vitamin K is calcium metabolism in your body. Problems with calcium metabolism can cause glutamate sensitivity, and excess oxalic acid production and circulation in your body. Vitamin K may work with calcium to heal leaky gut. It is also anti-inflammatory, a powerful anti-oxidant and helps to balance your insulin levels.

Most people are deficient in vitamin K (and its co-vitamin

Vitamin D) and it is highly likely that people with poor gut health will have very low levels of vitamin K because it is largely synthesised by probiotic gut bacteria. If you are going to take a supplement, take vitamin K2 and consume it with fat as it is fat-soluble and needs fat to be absorbed. Many vitamin K2 supplements are formulated from a wheat or soy base and contain glutamates and histamine. If you are sensitive to wheat or soy you could try finding a soy/wheat-free brand. If you are sensitive to glutamates and/or histamine start with a very small dose and build it up very slowly. I take a brand that is formulated from soy, but the packaging states that the product itself does not contain soy. When I first started taking it, I had a very strong glutamate reaction to it. I dropped the dose right down to the smallest pinch and after a couple of weeks the reaction subsided so I have been very slowly increasing the dose.

The recommended dose for vitamin K2 is between 45 mcg and 185 mcg daily for adults. If you are pregnant, are taking anti-coagulant medication or have experienced stroke, cardiac arrest, or are prone to blood clotting, you should not take vitamin K2 without first consulting your physician.

Biotin
Biotin is one of the B vitamins. I have read many reports of people finding it very helpful and I myself found that it reduced my symptoms especially those related to my skin. I experience almost no acne when I am taking daily doses of biotin. Biotin provides sulphate and has an anti-candida effect.

Be aware however, that biotin can cause digestive upset/nausea. Start with a low dose and build up. You may need to build up to quite high doses to see an impact (10,000mcg). Biotin has a low toxicity because it is a water-soluble vitamin and any excess is usually just excreted through urine, but it does deplete magnesium so you may need to take extra magnesium if you are taking biotin. Biotin may also stimulate hair growth, including facial hair growth. I found this was the case for me, and because I was uncomfortable with the excessive facial hair issues, I stopped taking biotin. I have thought about trying it again though at a lower dose.

Iron
Iron is needed to produce haemoglobin in our blood which carries oxygen around our body. Iron metabolism provides vital energy for our brain, muscles and immune system. Iron is needed for optimum immune system function. Iron is also necessary for normal cell function and in the making of some hormones and connective tissue. The best food sources of iron are red meat and eggs. Chicken and fish contain iron, but not as much as red meat. Wholegrains, potatoes, legumes and leafy greens are good sources of non-heme iron. Non-heme iron is not as well absorbed as heme iron. To boost absorption, eat non-heme iron sources with foods containing vitamin C.

If you cannot tolerate red meat and/or eggs or have digestive health issues that inhibit the absorption of nutrients (which is most of us with chemical and food intolerances) then it is likely that your iron levels are low. Iron deficiency is very common especially amongst women. Low iron levels may cause some symptoms that are the same as chemical intolerance symptoms such as irritability and fatigue. My daughter is generally much less tired and grumpy when she is taking a daily iron supplement.

Avoid taking iron supplements with tea, calcium or milk/dairy products as they will inhibit the iron from being absorbed. Iron is best absorbed on an empty stomach, however that can also increase the likelihood of it causing digestive upset or nausea. To reduce the risk of digestive upset you could break down the daily dose into 2 or 3 parts and take them over the course of the day rather than one large dose. Taking iron supplements between meals also prevents the possibility of the high iron intake inhibiting your absorption of zinc from foods. I personally find iron supplements energising so I prefer not to take them in the evening. Take only the recommended dose. Excess iron can cause gastric upset, nausea, constipation, abdominal pain, vomiting and faintness, and may act as an oxidant. Liquid supplements are generally less likely to cause constipation. Ferrous iron in dietary supplements is more bioavailable than ferric iron. Other forms of supplemental iron, such as heme iron polypeptides, carbonyl iron, iron amino-acid chelates, and polysaccharide-iron complexes, might have fewer gastrointestinal side effects than ferrous or ferric salts. It is wise to get your iron levels tested before taking a supplement. Ask for a blood test that evaluates your complete blood count (CBC), levels of serum ferritin, total iron-binding capacity, and/or transferrin.

Molybdenum
Molybdenum is needed for the sulphation detoxification process. A lack of molybdenum seems to cause an increase in the amount of sulphate lost through urine so a molybdenum supplement may help your body retain and recycle sulphate if your molybdenum levels are low. However, we only need trace amounts and be aware that excess molybdenum i.e., a supplement level of over 100mg a day, will reduce the functioning of the sulphation process.

Selenium
Selenium is essential for thyroid hormone metabolism, DNA repair and protection from oxidative damage and infection. It is critical to the optimum functioning of your immune system and liver, and your liver is a critical part of your body's

detoxification systems. Selenium is needed to form glutathione-based enzymes which link to and remove toxins. Along with magnesium and zinc, selenium may help protect glutamate receptors from excessive absorption.

Wholegrains and animal proteins such as fish, eggs, liver and fish and are the best food sources for those of us with chemical intolerances, but the amount of selenium in these sources may be low due to poor soil levels. In many countries the soil is deficient in selenium meaning that plants grown in that soil, and the animals that eat those plants, have low levels of selenium too as plants absorb minerals from soil.

If you are going to take a selenium supplement, take no more than the recommended daily amount as excess selenium can cause discoloured teeth, garlic breath, brittle or white blotchy nails, skin rashes, hair loss and a metallic taste in your mouth. Extremely high levels can cause kidney and heart failure. It would be a good idea to get your selenium and iodine levels checked before taking a supplement. If a selenium blood test shows that your level is above 1.6 mcrml/lt. there will probably be no advantage in taking extra, and taking a selenium supplement when your iodine levels are low can upset your thyroid function.

Vitamin B12
Vitamin B12 plays a key role in the normal functioning of your brain and nervous system and in the formation of your blood. It is also essential for the metabolism of fatty acids and amino acids in your body. Vitamin B12 also helps our body to absorb folic acid which facilitates the release of energy. Low B12 levels may restrict the activity of B12 related enzymes leading to elevated homocysteine levels.

The best food sources of vitamin B12 are red meat and eggs. Vitamin B12 is also found in fish, chicken and milk, but in lower levels. If you cannot tolerate red meat, eggs or dairy, or experience ongoing high levels of stress, or have digestive health issues that inhibit the absorption of nutrients (which is most of us with chemical and food intolerances) then it is likely that your vitamin B12 levels are low. It is wise to get a blood test of your vitamin B12 levels before taking a supplement.

L-Histidine
Histidine naturally binds and chelates certain metals in your body including zinc. Without enough histidine, zinc can remain unbound in your body producing prostaglandins that cause allergic responses and inflammation. Increasing your histidine level if it is low will cause zinc to be properly bound and excess excreted reducing allergic reaction responses, and it will reduce your body's production of histamine. Histidine also helps to chelate and remove toxic metals like mercury and cadmium.

You can get histidine from meat, dairy, kidney beans and eggs, but anyone with poor liver function will have difficulty synthesising histidine. Before taking a supplement, it is advisable to get your serum and urine amino acid levels checked to see if your histidine levels are low. Taking excess histidine may cause a deficiency of zinc (and nickel). If you take too much histidine you may experience the following symptoms:
- swollen membranes in your nose
- decreased sense of smell
- increased blood sugar
- constipation

It is advisable to take histidine with a low dose zinc supplement and B vitamins, especially vitamin B6.

Omega 3 Fatty Acids

EPA and DHA omega 3 fatty acids are anti-inflammatory and very beneficial. I have read of a study which found that regular intake of a fish oil supplement significantly reduced salicylate sensitivity. However, omega 3 supplements contain a number of elements which may be problematic. Fish oil supplements contain histamine and can also be contaminated with toxins such as mercury, other heavy metals and PCBs. Fish oil supplements usually also have some kind of anti-oxidant added and these are often problematic for those of us with chemical intolerances. Common additives include orange oil or rosemary extract, which may be high in salicylates and also likely to be problematic for those with histamine issues. Vitamin E (d-alpha Tocopherol) is another common additive, and could be made from petrochemicals or from refined soybean oil. Many fish oil supplements also contain added flavouring to disguise the fishy taste. I have found a couple of fish oil supplements that appear to be free of contaminants, flavourings and preservatives such as *Source Naturals Arctic Pure Omega-3 Fish Oil* and *Madre Labs Omega 3 Premium Fish Oil*, but these both still contain tocopherols and/or soy, and of course amines.

Some people suggest taking flaxseed or chia seed as an alternative source of omega 3. I wouldn't recommend this. Firstly, both flaxseed and chia are high in salicylates. I tried using ground chia in some gluten-free baked goods, but it gave me painful, inflamed joints every time, and then I found out it was a member of the mint family. Flaxseed and chia also contain the form of omega 3 known as alpha-linoleic acid (ALA). ALA is not equivalent to DHA or EPA in its biological effects, and needs to be converted to EPA in your body in order to be effective.

You can also buy omega 3 sourced from algae. However, seaweed is high in salicylates and sulphur, and also contains amines and glutamates. Moreover, algae-based supplements are likely to contain problematic anti-oxidants such as rosemary extract.

For most of us with chemical intolerances the best way to keep our omega 3 levels balanced is to keep our intake of refined cooking oils (polyunsaturated fats) to a minimum, and if possible, eat fresh fish at least 2-3 times a week. Grass-fed free-range beef, lamb and chicken also contain significant amounts of omega 3, but the meat from grain-fed animals raised in confined environments does not.

Calcium
Calcium is important for the formation of bones and teeth, and for muscle contraction, enzyme activity, nerve health and cell formation. It can also help promote restful sleep. For those of us who suffer from skin issues calcium increases moisture levels in the skin, improves the acid mantle, and reduces itching. As I eat virtually no dairy products, I thought that I would try a calcium supplement. I react to calcium citrate, and coral calcium, which is high in sulphur (and may also contain toxic aluminium and strontium), so I tried calcium carbonate. At first, I just added some to my toothpowder and that seemed to be alright so I started adding a ½ recommended dose to my breakfast. My skin, which had been relatively clear started breaking out in cystic acne and my eyes started to get irritated and felt oily and smeary. I sometimes felt like I was struggling to see things in focus. I had added it to some baking for my children, but it seemed to be causing them stomach upset and possibly constipation. When I did some more research, I learned that eye and stomach irritation and bowel upset are common side effects of calcium carbonate. Hence, I stopped taking it and giving it to my children and the symptoms cleared. I sprinkled the rest of the calcium carbonate in the container onto the garden.

Taking a calcium supplement can be problematic. The amino acid chelates known as citrate, aspartate and glutamate are often used as chelating agents in mineral supplements. These are suspected of containing or creating sufficient processed free glutamic acid to trigger MSG type reactions in sensitive people. In other words, if you are sensitive to glutamates, it is best to avoid chelated mineral supplements especially those labelled citrate, aspartate or glutamate. Also, if you eat a high calcium/dairy-rich diet or take calcium supplements or calcium-based antacids such as calcium carbonate (e.g., Tums), then be aware that taking significant amounts of sodium bicarbonate at the same time can cause milk-alkali syndrome resulting in metastatic calcification, kidney stones and kidney failure.

Although I experienced issues with the calcium carbonate supplement, I do seem to be able to take eggshell powder, which is natural calcium carbonate, without any noticeable problems. You can learn how to make this, how to get the most calcium you can from diet, and how to reduce lifestyle factors that cause the loss or mal-absorption of calcium in Step 3 - Diet: Avoid The Inflammatory 5: Dairy on page 68.

Appendices

EFT for Food Intolerances

The Emotional Freedom Technique (EFT) or Meridian Tapping is an energy healing protocol that involves using your fingers to tap on specific meridian or pressure points while stating or focusing on certain emotions or beliefs. It can be used both to release limiting or destructive emotions and beliefs, as well as to imprint positive ones. If you have not tried EFT before then you can go to The Tapping Solution website to learn how to do it.

The following EFT/Meridian Tapping script is the result of reading and personal tapping on this issue. Adding in the slow deep breathing as part of the EFT tapping helps to induce a meditative state which is more conducive to lettings things go and allowing your own specific issues concerning food intolerances to rise to the surface from your sub-conscious. If specific memories or thoughts do come up for you then tap on them with the normal EFT sequence as they arise and then return to the script.

You will need a piece of a food that you or your body responds to negatively i.e., that you are intolerant to. You can do one ingredient at a time or foods with multiple ingredients. My advice, and I have no scientific back-up for this, just experience, would be to start with single specific foods until you get experienced at the practice because it is easier to focus clearly on one specific object.

The EFT sequence below works through the process of releasing negative fears, beliefs and energy around food and eating, and then programming in positive beliefs that specific foods and foods in general are safe, allowed and good for us.

The tapping points have been abbreviated to:
IE = inner eye
OE = outer eye
UE = under eye
UN = under nose
C = chin
UA = under-arm (bra strap)
L = liver (front right of body just under your ribs)
TH = top of the head

EFT Sequence for Releasing Food Intolerances

IE   I choose to release all negative energy, fear, anger and tension from my belly (take a slow deep breath)

OE   I choose to release all negative energy, fear, anger and tension from my liver (take a slow deep breath)

UE   I choose to release all negative energy, fear, anger and tension from my kidneys (take a slow deep breath)

UN   I choose to release all negative energy, fear, anger and tension from my intestines (take a slow deep breath)

C   I choose to release all negative energy, fear, anger and tension from my belly (take a slow deep breath)

CB   I choose to release all negative energy, fear, anger and tension from my liver (take a slow deep breath)

UA   I choose to release all negative energy, fear, anger and tension from my kidneys (take a slow deep breath)

L   I choose to release all negative energy, fear, anger and tension from my intestines (take a slow deep breath)

TH   I choose to release all negative energy, fear, anger and tension from my belly (take a slow deep breath)

Now hold a small piece of the particular food you want to tap on in one hand and tap with the other. You can do one specific food at a time or something consisting of multiple ingredients. Look at the food while you are tapping so that both energy reactions in your body, physical skin reactions in your body, and psychological reactions in your brain are triggered.

IE   My body's reaction to this food (take a slow deep breath)

OE   My body's reaction to this food (take a slow deep breath)

UE   My body's reaction to this food (take a slow deep breath)

UN   My body's reaction to this food (take a slow deep breath)

C   My body's reaction to this food (take a slow deep breath)

CB   My body's reaction to this food (take a slow deep breath)

UA   My body's reaction to this food (take a slow deep breath)

L   My body's reaction to this food (take a slow deep breath)

TH   My body's reaction to this food (take a slow deep breath)

IE   I choose to release all programming from my body that sees this food as toxic (take a slow deep breath)

OE   I choose to release all programming from my body that sees this food as toxic (take a slow deep breath)

UE   I choose to release all programming from my body that sees this food as toxic (take a slow deep breath)

UN   I choose to release all programming from my body that sees this food as toxic (take a slow deep breath)

C   I choose to release all programming from my body that sees this food as toxic (take a slow deep breath)

CB   I choose to release all programming from my body that sees this food as toxic (take a slow deep breath)

UA   I choose to release all programming from my body that sees this food as toxic (take a slow deep breath)

L   I choose to release all programming from my body that sees this food as toxic (take a slow deep breath)

TH   I choose to release all programming from my body that sees this food as toxic (take a slow deep breath)

IE   I chose to release my fear of this food (breathe)
        OE   I choose to release all negative beliefs connected with this food (breathe)

UE   I choose to release all negative beliefs connected with food and eating (breathe)

UN   I choose to release the belief that I can't eat this food (breathe)

C   I choose to release the belief that this food is bad for me (breathe)

CB   I choose to release the belief that I am not allowed to eat this food (breathe)

UA   I chose to release my fear of this food (breathe)

L   I choose to release all negative beliefs connected with this food (breathe)

TH   I choose to release all negative beliefs connected with food and eating (breathe)

IE   I chose to believe that it is safe for me to eat this food (breathe)

OE   I choose to feel safe when I eat this food (breathe)
UE   I choose to feel safe and relaxed when I eat (breathe)
UN   I choose to believe that I am allowed to eat this food (breathe)
C   I choose to believe this food is good (breathe)
CB   I chose to believe that it is safe for me to eat this food (breathe)
S   I choose to feel safe when I eat this food (breathe)
L   I choose to believe that I can eat this food (breathe)
TH   I choose to feel safe and relaxed when I eat (breathe)

Resources

Support Groups/Forums
Food Intolerance Network Canterbury - finCant Yahoo Group
Fed Up.com – Food Intolerance Network Forum
Fed Up.com list of email support groups/yahoo groups
Salicylate Sensitivity.com Forum

Facebook:
Sue Dengate Failsafe Group
Beyond Failsafe – Biomed Chat
Food intolerance network NZ
Salicylate sensitivity

Recommended Products
Baking Soda/Sodium bicarbonate (edible)
Rob's Red Mill – I like this best for cleaning my teeth as it has a mild taste and smooth feel.

Brain Retraining
The Gupta Programme - guptaprogramme.com
Dynamic Neural Retraining System - retrainingthebrain.com

Cleaning
Baking Soda – in New Zealand you can buy sodium bicarbonate/baking soda in bulk from PGG Wrightson, Binn Inn and Bulk Barn stores

Ecostore – make a wide range of fragrance-free products which are also free of toxic chemicals and largely free of salicylates, glutamates, sulphur and amines (but not completely). I use and recommend their fragrance-free dishwash tablets, laundry soaker and handwash – ecostore.co.nz

Enjo microfiber cloths – enjo.com

Cookware
The Pampered Chef – pamperedchef.com
traditionalcook.com – buy toxic-free cookware online

Dental
The Water Flosser (appliance which uses only water to floss teeth)

Gobamboo.co.nz - bamboo toothbrushes

Food
Peas for Sprouting
Kings Seeds – kingsseeds.co.nz

Make-up
Andrea Rose - andrearose.com
Cleure - cleure.com
Immersion Pure Mineral Make-up
    immersioncosmetics.co.nz

Odor/Chemical Removal (from air)
Smelleze/No Odor – noodor.com – wide range of natural, non-toxic, re-usable products to remove odors and chemicals from the air. Products are formulated for specific situations e.g., paint odour removal, vehicle, vomit and chemical sensitivity.

Personal Care
Andrea Rose - andrearose.com
Cleure - cleure.com
Eco-store – ecostore.co.nz
Fed-Up website - fedup.com.au

Shoes
Soul Shoes – natural leather shoes, sandals, boots and bags - soulshoes.co.nz

Feelgoodz – natural rubber jandals/flip flops/sandals - feelgoodz.com

Zig Zag Jandals – rubber upper with foam undersole pad, available in New Zealand from Para Rubber and Hannahs

Supplements I have found beneficial
(Many of these can be obtained from www.iherb.com which is accessible in most countries.
Enzymedica Pro-bio probiotic
Nutricology Biotin 5000
Go Healthy Selenium
Go Healthy Vitamin D3
Go Healthy Vitamin K2
Eidon Ionic Minerals Zinc
Skybright Liquid Minerals – Iodine, Zinc, Iron, Selenium
Spatone 100% natural liquid iron supplement
Phenolgest by *Enzymedica*
Thorne Vitamin D + K2 (Thorne supplements contain no unnecessary fillers and no magnesium stearate. Information indicates that they are one of the highest quality supplement brands.)

Recommended Resources
Books and Web Pages
Change Your Diet and Change Your Life: Food Intolerance and Food Allergy Handbook by Sharla Race

Dr Rodney Ford – Dr Rodney Ford has written a number of books on the health issues that gluten consumption can cause: http://drrodneyford.com/about-us/dr-rodney-ford/books-by-dr-rodney-ford.html

Enzymes: Go With Your Gut by Karen DeFelice
I have read several books on using enzymes to aid health and this is by far the best. Easy and enjoyable to read,

comprehensive and up-to-date with clear, practical guidelines.

Fed Up: Understanding how food affects your child and what you can do about it by Sue Dengate
Fed Up is an informative and practical book and covers food lists and recipes for salicylate and amine intolerance well. However, if you also have a sulphur intolerance then most of the recipes are not relevant.

Good Health in the 21st Century by Dr Carole Hungerford

Karen Fischer – *The Eczema Diet* – www.jolieeskin.com
Karen Fischer writes extensively about the connection between salicylate intolerance and eczema

Natural Solutions for Food Allergies and Food Intolerances: Scientifically Proven Remedies for Food Sensitivities by Case Adams PhD

Pure Water: The Science of Water, Waves, Water Pollution, Water Treatment, Water Therapy and Water Ecology by Case Adams

The Paleo Approach: Reverse Autoimmune Disease and Heal Your Body by Sarah Ballantyne PhD. This book contains a substantial amount of thoroughly researched information on the connection between the food we eat and our biological function. It is a tome, but the information is clearly and attractively laid out making it easy to read and navigate.

What HIT me? Living with Histamine Intolerance by Genny Masterman

Why Isn't My Brain Working?: A Revolutionary Understanding of Brain Decline and Effective Strategies to Recover Your Brain's Health by Dr Datis Kharrazian. *Why Isn't My Brain Working?* Contains a lot of information on how food intolerance causes brain inflammation and what you can do to increase the health of your brain. Informative and practical.

Chemical-free Living
Debra Lynn Dadd: debralynndadd.com provides extensive lists of toxic-free products and information on toxin-free living.

Clean Water
Pure Water: The Science of Water, Waves, Water Pollution, Water Treatment, Water Therapy and Water Ecology by Case Adams
www.cleanairpurewater.com

Dental Floss
www.oilpulling.com

Diet
Information on digestive enzymes - enzymestuff.com
www.failsafediet.com
Fed Up by Sue Dengate and the corresponding website: fedup.com.au

Friendly Food by Anne Swain and the Royal Prince Albert Hospital (RPAH) Allergy Unit website

The Low Histamine Chef - Yasmina Ykelenstam's blog has a wealth of well researched information regarding Histamine Intolerance and mast cell disorders. Her free ebook "Yasmina's Top 10 Food Re-introduction Tips" is very interesting. The following post in particular provides a thorough basic overview of what histamine intolerance is including how to diagnose it, facts about what you can and cannot eat, what helps lower histamine levels and what to be wary of: Dr Joneja interview

Millhouse Integrative Medical Centre: millhousemedical.co.nz

Under the resources section on this website are a list of factsheets prepared by Dr Ric Coleman including ones on low amine diet, low salicylate diet, relaxation and breathing. You can view these for free as a pdf. Millhouse Medical is located in Howick, Auckland, New Zealand and may be an option if you live in that area and are looking for a medical practitioner familiar with chemical sensitivities.

Salicylate Sensitivity.com

Truth in Labeling.org has thorough lists on sources of MSG (for those sensitive to glutamates)

Dietitians
Failsafe: there is a list of Failsafe aware dietitians and other health practitioners available on the fedup.com.au website.

Biomed: The Bio-Balance website has information about biochemical and nutritional based treatment of health issues such as ADHD, behavioural disorders, learning disorders and mental disorders. Many people with chemical intolerance issues have found this treatment helpful. You can find more information and a list of biomedical practitioners at www.bioblance.org.au

Dry Body Brushing & Self-Massage
Dry body brushing - www.bodecare.com
Facial and whole body massage for lymphatic drainage videos on Youtube

Frequency Generators
The Ultimate Zapper: http://zap.intergate.ca/
Hulda Clark research: www.drclark.net

Pea Sprouts
Is Food Making You Sick – Natural Sources of DAO

Vickerstaff Health Services Inc Factsheet Diamine Oxidase from Pea Seedlings

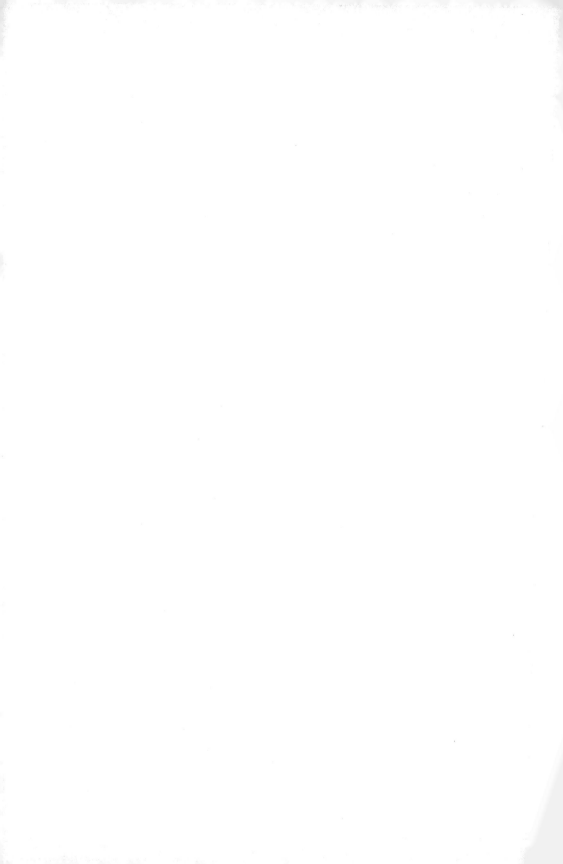